Everything

You Need to Know About the

Menopause

A comprehensive guide to surviving – and
thriving! – during this turbulent life stage

Ellen Phillips

RODALE

This edition first published in the UK in 2004 by
Rodale International Ltd
7–10 Chandos Street
London W1G 9AD
www.rodalestore.co.uk

Printed and bound in Italy by Rotolito Lombrda s.p.a. using acid-free paper from sustainable sources

1 3 5 7 9 8 6 4 2

A CIP record for this book is available from the British Library
ISBN 1-4050-6723-3

Notice

This book is intended as a reference volume only, not as a medical manual. The information given here is designed to help you make informed decisions about your health. It is not intended as a substitute for any treatment that may have been prescribed by your doctor. If you suspect that you have a medical problem, we urge you to seek competent medical help.

Beginning on page 331, you will find safe use guidelines for supplements, herbs or essential oils recommended in this book that will help you use these remedies safely and wisely.

Mention of specific companies, organizations or authorities in this book does not imply endorsement by the publisher, nor does mention of specific companies, organizations or authorities imply that they endorse this book.

Internet addresses and telephone numbers given in this book were accurate at the time it went to press.

Portions of this book have been adapted from material that has appeared in *Prevention* magazine and in the following Rodale books: *Age Erasers for Women; Extraordinary Togetherness; Get Well/Stay Well; New Choices in Natural Healing for Women; Doctors Book of Home Remedies*, revised edition; *Doctors Book of Home Remedies for Managing Menopause; Doctors Book of Home Remedies for Seniors; Doctors Book of Home Remedies for Women; Natural Prescriptions; Natural Hormone Solutions; Nature's Medicine; Women's Book of Healing Herbs; Women's Edge: Growing Younger; Women's Edge: Natural Hormones; Women's Edge: Natural Calm; Women's Edge: Energy for Everything; Women's Edge: The Inner Journey; Women's Wisdom That Works*

Prevention is the world's largest-circulation health magazine: it brings up-to-date, thoroughly researched and fact-checked health information to its more than 11 million readers every month. *Everything You Need to Know About the Menopause*, written by the Editors of *Prevention*, draws on the wisdom and expertise of the magazine's large team of medical advisors and other healthcare experts.

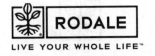

CONTENTS

MENOPAUSE:
NEW DIRECTIONS

No TWO WOMEN GO THROUGH MENOPAUSE IN EXACTLY THE same way. One experiences hot flushes that will melt steel; others suffer chills – or one of 50 other possible mental or physical changes. In the past, most women confronted by menopause had two choices – suffer the symptoms (usually in silence), or take a hormone tablet. But then along came the startling findings of the Women's Health Initiative Study in the US, which concluded that the potential health hazards of using Prempro, a type of hormone replacement therapy containing oestrogen and progesterone, outweighed its benefits. Subsequent research into other forms of HRT confirmed these findings, and when the National Toxicology Program in the US classified oestrogen as a carcinogen, women – and their doctors – around the world were thrown into turmoil. What's more, a study in the 9 August 2003 issue of *The Lancet*, involving more than a million women in the UK, found strong evidence that use of combination HRT is associated with a substantially greater risk of breast cancer. Women who are nearing menopause or are in the midst of it are asking themselves, 'What do I do now?' And they're realizing that there are no easy answers.

In some ways, the flurry of publicity surrounding the study results has been a good thing. For one, it's brought menopause out of the closet and into the open. When mainstream newspapers and magazines run a cover story on menopause, women find it easier to talk about it – with one another, with their families, with their doctors – rather than suffering in silence, wondering what on earth is happening or is going to happen to them, and fearing the future. For another, it's forced the medical profession to take alternative therapies seriously. Doctors are telling their patients about soya for hormonal imbalances, black cohosh for relief of menopausal symptoms, yoga for stress relief, and a host of other options, as well as discussing all the conventional treatments. Finally, menopause's unlikely entry into the spotlight has given women the opportunity to look at it in new ways. Rather than viewing menopause as a disease to be 'cured' – or at least postponed – by medical treatment, or as the gateway to old age, women are starting to see it as an empowering life stage. Bestsellers like Christiane Northrup's *The Wisdom of Menopause* and Mary Jane Minkin's pioneering *What Every Woman Needs to Know About Menopause* have paved the way for this very positive change.

But one thing is certain: more than ever, perimenopausal, menopausal and postmenopausal women have to take their lives and their treatment into their own hands, because virtually every lifestyle change you make today will affect your health and vitality for the rest of your life. These critical changes can make the difference between a slow decline into helplessness and the best years of your life. And that's why we've written this book – to give you the guidance you need to make the best choices for you. We've consulted the top experts in the field, drawn from the latest research, and sifted through all the conflicting data to bring you the definitive guide for what could be the beginning of the most exciting, fulfilling time of your life. Whether you're 35 and just experiencing a few odd symptoms, facing menopause and wondering about your options, or on the other side and looking ahead, this book will give you a wealth of doctor-approved ways to manage your symptoms, your diet, your moods, your stress levels, your looks – even your sex life!

Turn to our extensive 'Menopause Symptom Solver' to look up symptoms as you experience them – and for every menopausal woman, the range and severity of symptoms will vary – and find out all the recommended conventional and alternative treatments and preventives for each symptom. Chapters on conventional and alternative treatment options allow you to read in-depth about each treatment, its advantages and drawbacks, when and how it works best and what can enhance its performance, as well as which remedies should never be combined. Another helpful feature is 'Straight Talk About the Menopause', answering women's most frequently asked questions.

Menopause confronts women with unique challenges. Our bodies present us with a wide range of often debilitating symptoms, our moods and emotions seem out of our control, we begin gaining midbody weight for no reason, we may lose interest in sex, and new sags and wrinkles mysteriously pop up on our faces and bodies every day, adding the spectre of old age to all the other changes. *Everything You Need to Know About the Menopause* presents a comprehensive programme to help women triumph over each of these challenges, conquer the stress that menopause often piles on to an already hectic lifestyle, and emerge attractive, centred and vibrantly healthy. Please join us for the journey!

Ellen Phillips, Editor

PART

1

What's Going On?

Your body's changing, medical recommendations are changing, your moods and emotions are changing – suddenly, it seems like *everything's* changing! In this section, we'll tell you what to expect before, during and after the menopause, so none of the possible symptoms will take you by surprise. And we'll give you our recommendations for getting a fast grip on the situation, minimizing discomfort and laying the foundation for vibrant good health, good looks and good times for the rest of your life.

Chapter

1

WHAT TO EXPECT: A MENOPAUSE TIMELINE

If you're gearing up to go through the menopause, or have already done so, you must know you're not alone. Menopause has come out of the closet in a big way, as the huge wave of Baby Boomer females who took control of their reproductive health during the 1970s and beyond are now taking control of their post-reproductive years.

Unlike our mothers, most of us never have defined ourselves solely as mothers or wives. So it's only natural that we take that expansive sense of self with us into our later years. We are not buying the traditional role of 'little old lady'. In fact, we may be the first generation of grandmothers who pump iron to prevent osteoporosis and use testosterone to boost sex drive.

In the past, menopause and the years beyond were often painted as a bleak picture – a time of depression, low energy and terminal grumpiness – mostly because women didn't see their doctors about it unless they had serious symptoms. But more recently, women's experience shows that the menopause is *not* all negative for most women. If it seems to be really bad for you, you'd be wise to discuss it with your doctor. A good doctor can

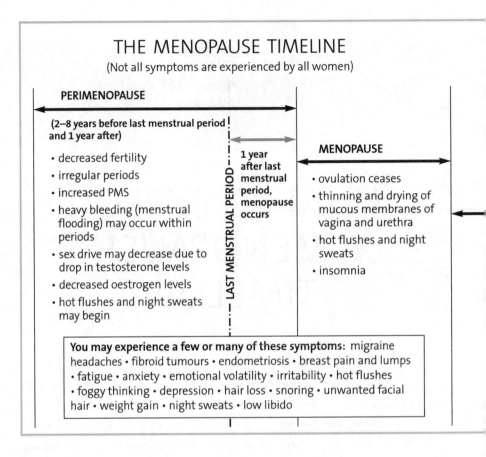

THE MENOPAUSE TIMELINE
(Not all symptoms are experienced by all women)

PERIMENOPAUSE

(2–8 years before last menstrual period and 1 year after)

- decreased fertility
- irregular periods
- increased PMS
- heavy bleeding (menstrual flooding) may occur within periods
- sex drive may decrease due to drop in testosterone levels
- decreased oestrogen levels
- hot flushes and night sweats may begin

LAST MENSTRUAL PERIOD

1 year after last menstrual period, menopause occurs

MENOPAUSE

- ovulation ceases
- thinning and drying of mucous membranes of vagina and urethra
- hot flushes and night sweats
- insomnia

You may experience a few or many of these symptoms: migraine headaches • fibroid tumours • endometriosis • breast pain and lumps • fatigue • anxiety • emotional volatility • irritability • hot flushes • foggy thinking • depression • hair loss • snoring • unwanted facial hair • weight gain • night sweats • low libido

establish which of your problems are related to the menopause and which aren't, and provide help in both cases.

More recently, the menopause has also been romanticized as a time of new wisdom, freedom and inner strength, and that's certainly possible for those who use this time of transition for self-growth. (It doesn't happen automatically!) The groundbreaking book on postmenopausal empowerment is Christiane Northrup's *The Wisdom of Menopause*. We strongly recommend it.

But even as the menopause has finally come out of the closet and started to take on positive overtones, it has become more challenging, too. In the past, women were encouraged by their doctors to normalize their hormone levels and ward off menopausal symptoms by taking oestrogen

POSTMENOPAUSE

- skin becomes thin
- cholesterol levels increase
- good cholesterol (HDL) decreases
- bones become more brittle; risk of osteoporosis and fractures increases
- muscles lose tone
- increased risk of heart disease
- hot flushes may continue
- increased risk of cancer

The symptoms in this timeline may look intimidating – even frightening. It's important to remember that some women go through menopause without experiencing any symptoms, and most symptoms can be prevented or treated. (We'll show you how in the rest of this book!) The purpose of this timeline is to act as a checkpoint for you, so if you experience symptoms, you'll be able to identify them instantly and then take the appropriate action.

or oestrogen/progesterone in tablet form, a treatment called hormone replacement therapy (HRT). Many doctors are now more reluctant to prescribe HRT in light of the recent study by the National Institutes of Health in the US that linked hormone therapy to cancer, as well as the inclusion of oestrogen replacement therapy on the US government list of cancer-causing agents. UK cancer organizations were quick to follow suit, listing oestrogen as a potential carcinogen for all women. (See 'New Directions' on page 5 for more about these findings.) Because of the potential dangers of hormone therapy, all women need to take a more active role in managing their menopause, both to prevent future problems like osteoporosis and weight gain and to minimize or eliminate unpleasant symptoms like hot flushes. And that's what this book is about.

In this chapter, we'll present a timeline of facts about the menopause and the years before and after. The menopause is inevitable and, as with everything else that happens in life, it's up to you to make the best of it, with both good self-care and good medical care. Every woman is different, but most can fit themselves somewhere into this time frame. Keep in mind that while medicine creates premenopausal, perimenopausal and post-menopausal categories, women's symptoms don't always fit so neatly into that scheme. So read through this short chapter and see the whole range of symptoms and experiences that can occur during these transitional years. Then, whatever you're experiencing, you'll know where it fits in the overall menopause picture.

What Is the Menopause, Anyway?

Even the word 'menopause' is used loosely. The term actually refers to only *one day* in your life – the 365th day from the date of your last period. (The time after that is called postmenopause.) It's only in retrospect that you know you have reached the menopause, and plenty – in fact, most – women have lots of 'false starts'. They may go for months without a period, and then get one – usually while on holiday.

This demarcation is medically important because menopause means your body no longer produces enough oestrogen to support a menstrual cycle. Doctors are much more suspicious of irregular uterine bleeding after menopause – during perimenopause (two to eight years before your last menstrual period and one year after), it's a given.

The average age of 'natural' menopause for Caucasian women (that is, not induced by surgery, chemotherapy or radiation) in the West is 51, and that figure hasn't changed much over the past few centuries. The normal range is 46 to 54. But some women reach the menopause in their thirties, and a few in their sixties. Women who smoke tend to reach the menopause a year or two earlier than nonsmokers. Overweight women tend to have a later menopause because body fat can convert some hormone precursors into oestrogen. (This higher oestrogen level also puts overweight women at increased risk for breast cancer.) Thin women tend to have a harder time of it at menopause, and are at higher risk for osteoporosis, than women with some extra body fat.

IS IT REALLY THE MENOPAUSE?

The only way to know for sure if you're in the perimenopause transition, or if you have reached the menopause itself, is through a visit to your doctor. He or she will rule out pregnancy or serious health problems like uterine cancer and can take a blood test to assess your oestrogen levels.

The most reliable test measures the level of follicle-stimulating hormone (FSH), a hormone secreted by the pituitary gland to stimulate oestrogen production. As the ovaries' oestrogen production decreases, the pituitary gland increases production of FSH. Levels of 30 to 40 mIU/mL (milli international units per millilitre) or above mean you've reached menopause. Levels from 10 to near 30 mean there's still partial ovarian function.

Even FSH levels, however, can sometimes be misleading. They tend to fluctuate from month to month during perimenopause. To confirm whether you're in perimenopause, your doctor should review not only your FSH results but also your medical history and the physical and emotional changes you're experiencing (irregular periods, hot flushes, and so on).

Some doctors won't do the FSH test unless you seem too young to be entering menopause. They'll simply assume on the basis of your symptoms that you're menopausal. If you believe yourself to have reached the menopause and want to make sure, ask your doctor to check your FSH levels if he or she doesn't volunteer to do so.

What Causes the Menopause?

The answer to this question is a simple one: our ovaries. Women depend on their ovaries to produce most of the oestrogen in their bodies. Ovaries also produce progesterone, a hormone that is less understood than oestrogen but that also has whole-body effects. (A recent study shows that just like oestrogen, progesterone can help reduce the incidence of hot flushes and help you sleep better.) Ovaries even produce small amounts of androgen hormones – the male stuff that fuels sex drive in both men and women. Unfortunately, our ovaries have a lifespan that's shorter than our current life expectancy. They tend to conk out about 25–30 years before the rest of our bodies.

The ovaries' manufacture of oestrogen and progesterone is dependent on a complex network of other hormones, including follicle–stimulating hormone (FSH) and luteinizing hormone (LH), both secreted by the brain's pituitary gland. Hormone production also depends on the ability of the ovaries to mature and release a ripe egg. The maturing egg 'sac', called the follicle, secretes oestrogen. After the egg is released, the empty egg sac, called the corpus luteum, secretes progesterone.

Lots of things start working against our ovaries as we age. First, an accelerated depletion of eggs from the ovaries begins somewhere between ages 35 and 40. Many eggs die off during a cycle, and sometimes more than one ripens during a cycle – hence the higher incidence of twins for women in their thirties than in their twenties. The ovaries also become less responsive to the stimulating effects of FSH and LH, so levels of these hormones start to rise. You have fewer cycles in which you ovulate, and because progesterone is produced in the corpus luteum, after ovulation you might see a drop-off of progesterone first, while oestrogen levels remain closer to normal. This condition, called oestrogen dominance, is the reason some alternative doctors have recommended supplemental progesterone to women during the perimenopausal years.

Finally, there are no more eggs to be released, so there is no egg follicle to secrete oestrogen or, after an egg is released, to switch over and secrete progesterone. Progesterone drops to very low levels, but the ovaries continue to make declining amounts of oestrogen for a few years after menopause. Eventually, however, they stop functioning as endocrine glands. The adrenal glands, however, continue to make small amounts of sex hormone precursors, such as DHEA (dehydroepiandros-terone). These can be converted to oestrogen (or testosterone) in the fat tissues of the body.

In addition to oestrogen, your blood levels of testosterone, the 'hormone of desire', drop by about 50 per cent between ages 20 and 40, and then more slowly trail the decline of oestrogen after menopause.

Perimenopause: the Start of It All

The term perimenopause was coined only recently. *Peri-*, by the way, means 'near' or 'around', so perimenopause simply means 'around the time of menopause'. It now officially refers to the two to eight years preceding menopause and the year after menopause. So, for most women, peri-menopause begins sometime in the mid-forties, but it can begin as early as the mid- to late thirties. (See 'Too Young for Menopause?' below.)

Perimenopause is a time of hormone fluctuations that may begin fairly subtly, then slowly become more exaggerated as a woman approaches menopause. Oestrogen levels may go as high as those seen during early pregnancy, only to drop and stay low for some time. Health conditions influenced by unstable hormone levels are likely to worsen during this time. These include migraine headaches, fibroid tumours, endometriosis, PMS, irregular menstrual cycles and fibrocystic breast disorder.

Women also usually have their first hot flushes and night sweats during this time – and may at first wonder, 'What on earth is this?!' Some women complain of fatigue; of emotional swings, anxiety or irritability; of foggy thinking; or of just plain not feeling right. We all need to realize that the feelings we're having at this time aren't simply emotional – they're the result of actual hormonal changes in our bodies. Even the brain has receptor sites for oestrogen – and feels deprived when it doesn't get the hormone in the amounts it expects.

For many women, perimenopause is a rougher ride than post-menopause. Luckily, many of the lifestyle changes we suggest in this book are helpful for these symptoms. Natural alternatives – such as black

TOO YOUNG FOR THE MENOPAUSE?

Menopause before the age of 40, technically called premature ovarian failure, is rare. Only about 1 per cent of women go through menopause before the age of 40. It tends to run in families, and tests often show that these women have developed an immune response to their bodies' own ovarian tissue. There also seems to be an association between premature ovarian failure and other autoimmune diseases, such as type 1 diabetes, thyroiditis (inflammation of the thyroid gland) and rheumatoid arthritis. The bottom line is that if you're in your thirties and experiencing signs of menopause, you should get your oestrogen and follicle-stimulating hormone measured. And get a thyroid-stimulating hormone (TSH) test as part of your check-up.

cohosh, soya foods and progesterone cream – can also make a big differ-ence to women during this time. Some doctors will also give women low-dose birth control pills to help control erratic hormone levels. And also, luckily, over time our bodies adjust to lower hormone levels so that by the time we're postmenopausal, some symptoms will have started to subside. But meanwhile, if you're experiencing unpleasant symptoms, check them out in Chapter 7, look up the recommended conventional and alternative treatments we recommend, and discuss with your doctor those that make sense to you.

Postmenopause: When It's Finally Over

Once you've gone a full year without periods, you are considered to be in the postmenopausal phase of your life. Your ovaries no longer pro-duce enough oestrogen and progesterone to support an ovulation cycle.

But far from it being the beginning of the end, many women see the time after menopause as a new beginning. In survey after survey women consistently report that their postmenopausal years are the most fulfilling and happiest of their lives. In one survey, by the Social Issues Research Centre in Oxford, 65 per cent of women between the ages of 50 and 64 said they felt happier than before the menopause. In the US, close to 80 per cent of women say that cessation of menstruation came as a relief. More than half say that reaching menopause was a positive turning point in their lives. They report having more time and energy to focus on hobbies, rela-tionships and other interests. And three out of four made some type of health-related improvement, such as finally stopping smoking. And that's all for the best since most women are postmenopausal for about one-third of their lives.

Symptoms linked to hormonal instability tend to diminish as we reach menopause, so migraines, PMS and endometriosis will tend to improve. Hot flushes will usually continue for a few years after the menopause, but they will gradually fade away.

Still, even if you have no immediate obvious symptoms as a result of your having reached menopause, over time you most definitely will have phys-ical changes, as a result of both diminishing hormone levels and ageing.

HORMONE THERAPY
FOR YOUR HUSBAND?

Picture an advertisement like this: a group of men are sitting around watching the big match, drinking a few beers, when one of them pipes up: 'I haven't been feeling myself lately. My doctor thinks I might need to go on HRT. I'm not sure what to do.'

A big, burly man named Dave comes back with: 'I know how you feel, Al. But since I've been on testosterone, I feel great! I'm vibrant, and my sex life has never been better!' The men raise their glasses in raucous approval.

This scene might not be so far-fetched. Male hormone therapy is available now and is expected to grow in popularity in the coming years.

The main hormone in male HRT is testosterone, says Keith Gordon, an expert in reproductive medicine.

As with oestrogen in women, testosterone starts to decline during a man's forties. Early on, testosterone deficiency presents itself as general malaise, depression and, perhaps, muscle weakness, Dr Gordon says. As the decline progresses, it can affect sexual function and, in the long-term, speed up osteoporosis. To ward off all these troubles, a man can take supplemental testosterone.

But just as with our hormone therapy, he'll have to weigh the benefits against the risks. In a man's case, supplemental testosterone could bring on benign prostatic hyperplasia, a condition in which the prostate grows larger and pushes against the urethra or bladder, blocking the normal flow of urine. If a man has the early stages of prostate cancer, testosterone could also speed the cancer's growth, Dr Gordon says.

You'll have thinning and drying of the mucous membranes of the vagina and urethra, which can set the stage for painful intercourse or urinary incontinence. You'll have gradual thinning of the skin, as well as slowly rising total cholesterol levels and a drop in the 'good' stuff – HDL cholesterol. You're likely to lose bone mass and muscle tone, especially if you don't exercise.

Some of these effects take decades to appear, but they do appear sooner or later in most women. These things are also very treatable, both with lifestyle changes and, if necessary, with drugs. Women who choose not to use hormone replacement therapy (HRT) to keep their bones strong, for instance, can do resistance training or take a bone-saving drug – a number of them are now on the market. Even some forms of HRT can be used selectively to reduce symptoms without much risk. One example is Estring, a vaginal ring that delivers a tiny amount (about 2 mg per day) of oestrogen to prevent vaginal dryness and atrophy and that can also help maintain the urethra. Its systemic effects are minimal. Women whose main complaint is loss of sex drive may find that a little testosterone cream applied to the clitoris provides the boost they need. (For details, see Chapter 6.)

Fewer than half of postmenopausal women took oestrogen before the recent studies implicating it in heart disease and cancer, and these days, with the bad press hormone therapy is receiving, even fewer are likely to take it, or at least to take it in its most commonly prescribed forms – Premarin, Premique and Prempak-C. Using no hormone therapy does make things harder for a woman. There's no easy way to make up for the fact that our bodies have run out of oestrogen. But there are ways to compensate – they include alternative therapies like soya foods and phyto-oestrogen-containing herbs, exercise and other lifestyle changes. We have literally hundreds of suggestions to help you. This book is designed to help you put it all together and have an easy menopause and a vibrant, healthy life once it's over.

PART

2

Looking Good, Feeling Great

The menopause is a time of transition, with day-to-day changes and symptoms that can last for years. But life doesn't screech to a halt – and neither should you. In this section, we'll show you how to live life to the fullest, minimizing negative changes (such as weight gain and hair loss) while discovering positive changes that will dramatically improve your life.

THE MENOPAUSE
EATING PLAN

THERE ARE PLENTY OF REASONS TO CHANGE THE WAY YOU EAT AS you approach the menopause. If you don't, you'll start gaining weight – even if you're eating the way you always did in the past. The foods you eat – or don't eat – can also increase or minimize menopausal symptoms, from hot flushes to bloating and wind. And foods are also key weapons in the fight against the major postmenopausal diseases: cancer, osteoporosis and heart disease.

With all this in mind, we've developed an eating plan that will help you to combat weight gain, menopausal symptoms and diseases. And it will help you look and feel great. We'll start with our core strategy: eating five or six mini-meals a day, rather than two or three biggies. (Find out why this works in the next section, 'Mini-Meals Fight "Menopause Midriffs"'.) Then, in 'Eating for an Easier Menopause' on page 24, we'll tell you about the menopause superfoods, the ones that promote overall radiant health and energy while reducing menopausal symptoms. Finally, we'll give you the latest recommendations on foods that fight disease in 'Cutting Your Cancer Risk' on page 43, 'Give Your Bones a Break from Osteoporosis' on page 46 and 'Heading Off Heart Disease' on page 50.

Food is one of the most basic, easiest and cheapest healthcare options available. Making clever food choices now can help you breeze through menopause, and keep you looking good and feeling great in your post-menopausal years.

Mini-meals Fight 'Menopause Midriffs'

The heart of our Menopause Eating Plan is mini-meals. There are four great reasons that mini-meals are the right choice for menopausal women. First, they help minimize mid-life weight gain. Second, eating small meals at regular intervals helps control the unpleasant digestive symptoms of menopause, including bloating, wind and diarrhoea. Third, eating frequent mini-meals gives you the steady supply of fuel you need to stay calm, focused and energetic all day, freed at last from the soar-and-crash seesaw caused by large, infrequent meals. And fourth, because you're never ravenous, you can make the food choices you'll need to stay healthy and vibrant, rather than panic in your hunger and grab the first high-fat, high-sugar energy booster you can lay your hands on.

Scientific research supports the mini-meal concept. Some studies have suggested that eating five or six smaller meals a day is better for you than eating the traditional three square meals, and can make it easier to control your weight, particularly as you age. Menopause specialists also support the idea of mini-meals.

To show you how it works, here's a tale of two menopause-age dieters on a typical day.

Woman number one is a mini-meal muncher. She breakfasts each morning on some cereal and orange juice, then heads off to work. About mid-morning she takes a break and gets a plain bagel to nibble on while she works. A few hours later she stops for lunch – a sandwich and some salad. By late afternoon she's having a snack of rice cakes. After work she heads home and whips up some grilled fish and a small potato for dinner. Later, when her chores are done, she sits down to watch TV and snacks on low-fat yoghurt and some grapes. Then it's time for bed.

Woman number two is a calorie watcher. She's out the door in the morning without any breakfast, and ignores her hunger pangs until lunch.

Finally, it's lunchtime. She picks at a small salad and then ignores her hunger all afternoon. About 5 pm, she heads home, polishes off a nice dinner, watches some TV and heads for bed.

Who's going to be the winner at losing?

Woman number one.

Why More Is Best

You'd think skipping meals would result in eating fewer calories, which in turn would result in less body fat. But your body doesn't work that way. It actually burns fat more effectively when you eat small amounts of food more often. In fact, scientists have discovered that eating four to six small meals a day actually helps to speed up your fat-burning system. Here's why.

- If you bypass breakfast and skimp on lunch, you're going to overload at dinner. 'After an all-day fast, the body is ravenous and you end up doubling the quantity of food you eat,' says Diane Grabowski-Nepa, a nutritionist. Too much food at any one time is more than your body can handle, and encourages fat storage. Plus, your body is more efficient at storing fat in the evening than earlier in the day, when you're more active. So if you overeat at dinner, more calories get stored as fat than, say, if you overeat at breakfast.

- Skipping meals can slow your metabolism by as much as 5 per cent. That's because an empty stomach makes your brain think your body is starving, so it turns down its calorie-burning thermostat in an effort to live longer off its stored fat. On the other hand, when you eat small meals all day long, your stomach never gets a chance to be empty, thus keeping your metabolism purring along.

- When you eat a big meal, such as a huge dinner, your body produces insulin, which stimulates an enzyme called lipoprotein lipase, or LPL. LPL opens up the door of fat cells, which can expand quite easily, and lets those lipids settle in. The more insulin you have, the more those fat cells can hold. High insulin levels also stimulate appetite, which makes you want to eat more. On the other hand, when you eat small meals all day long, you never experience the insulin surge that larger meals create.

MINI-MEAL MENU SAMPLER

It can be a little daunting to work out how to eat all day and still lose weight, so we asked Anne Dubner, a nutritionist, to put together some daily menus to show how satisfying mini-meals can be.

The trick to losing weight on mini-meals, she says, is to listen to your stomach. Eat when you start feeling a little hungry – don't wait until you're famished – and stop as soon as your hunger goes away, not when you're stuffed. That way, you'll stay satisfied all day. Here are three days' worth of menus to get you started.

DAY ONE

Breakfast: Half a wholewheat bread roll with puréed roasted peppers mixed with reduced-fat or fat-free cream cheese, a 240-ml (8-fl oz) glass of fat-free milk, and 75 g (2½ oz) of blueberries

Snack: The other half of the bread roll with roasted peppers

Lunch: Half a turkey sandwich (made with turkey breast, sliced tomato and lettuce) and a mixed garden salad with 1 tablespoon of reduced-fat dressing

Snack: The other half of the sandwich

Dinner: 300 g (10 ½ oz) of pasta primavera (made with fusilli or penne pasta, frozen mixed vegetables, garlic, Parmesan cheese and 1 tablespoon of olive oil) and a slice of bread topped with 1 teaspoon of reduced-fat margarine mixed with 1 teaspoon each of crushed fresh garlic and grated Parmesan cheese

Snack: An oatmeal raisin biscuit

DAY TWO

Breakfast: One slice of raisin bread with 1 tablespoon of peanut butter and a 120-ml (4-fl oz) glass of orange juice

Snack: A reduced-fat dried fruit bar and a 240-ml (8-oz) glass of fat-free milk

Lunch: Half a chicken salad pitta sandwich (made with low-fat, cubed cooked chicken, toasted walnuts, raisins, small grapes and honey) and 125 g (4½ oz) of raw vegetables such as baby carrots and celery

Snack: The other half of the sandwich

Dinner: Cheese quesadilla (made with a flour tortilla, 2 tablespoons of grated reduced-fat Cheddar cheese, 1½ teaspoons of chopped canned green chilli peppers, 1½ teaspoons of sliced black olives and salsa, chilli powder and sliced spring onions to taste) with 90 g (3 oz) of white rice mixed with 2 tablespoons of salsa

Snack: 230 g (8 oz) of fat-free flavoured yoghurt with two oatcakes

DAY THREE

Breakfast: An English muffin with one scrambled egg, a small orange and a 240-ml (8-fl oz) glass of fat-free milk

Snack: A sandwich made with half a banana and 1 tablespoon of peanut butter

Lunch: A small Greek salad (made with chopped tomatoes, cucumbers, sweet red peppers and onions, with feta cheese and a dressing of lemon juice and olive oil with oregano and garlic) and a small pitta bread

Snack: Six crackers with tuna salad (made with tuna, 1 tablespoon of reduced-fat mayonnaise and a squirt of lemon juice)

Dinner: Potato skins (made with one quartered baked potato, 60 g (2 oz) of grated reduced-fat Cheddar cheese, some spring onions or chives and paprika) with 90g (3 0z) of steamed broccoli

Snack: 3 handfuls of popcorn

- Spreading your daily calories over four meals or more can help you to dampen your appetite by keeping food in your stomach at all times. Instead of always feeling deprived, you always feel full, so you don't binge.

- Your stomach expands and contracts with food load, and apparently it loses its tone when repeatedly pushed to the max. So once your stomach is overstretched, it takes more food to satisfy you, according to studies by scientists at the obesity research centre at St Luke's–Roosevelt Hospital Center in New York. Eating small amounts of food all day doesn't stretch the stomach, so you feel full more quickly.

Mini-meal Magic

Ready to give it a try? Think variety. Continue to eat from all the food groups – grains, fruit, vegetables, dairy and protein – throughout the day. But you don't need to balance your intake of food groups at every meal as you did when you were eating three meals. Instead, you want to achieve balance over the course of an entire day, which means about eight grains, three or four fruits, four vegetables, two or three dairy products and five lean meats or other protein foods each day. Here's the best advice from experts for getting into the mini-meal mindset.

Give your regular meals the split. Try dividing what you eat for breakfast, lunch and dinner in half to create six meals, suggests nutritionist Anne Dubner. If you usually eat a bagel for breakfast, for example, eat half when you get up and the other half later. If you have a sandwich for lunch, eat the halves at two different times. That way, you won't spend any more time preparing food.

Watch the fat and the portions. In determining your daily intake, it's important to keep your eye on those two waist-expanding monsters, fat and calories. While fat reduction is the most important priority for good health and weight loss, you don't want calories to fall too low or climb too high.

Eat 'fight fat' foods. That means foods high in fibre and low in fat and added sugar – things like fruit, vegetables and wholegrain bread. Avoid empty-calorie snacks, like doughnuts.

Select a serving. Favour foods that are already portioned into individual servings, like a baked potato, a container of yoghurt or a bagel. Eating a set portion ensures that you'll stop when you're full (or nearly full) because you'll run out of food, says Michele Harvey, a diabetes expert and nutritionist.

MAKING THE CHANGE TO MINI-MEALS

Because she was overweight and diabetic, Anita Beattie's doctor gave her a harsh ultimatum: 'Enter a hospital programme to lose weight or don't come back to see me because you are wasting my time.' That push was just the encouragement Anita needed to drop the extra 16 kg (2½ st) that she was lugging around and, with her doctor's guidance, to taper off the insulin that she used to control her diabetes.

'My doctor put me in the hospital for four days to teach me enough about diet and exercise so that when I left the hospital, I could carry out these lessons on my own,' Anita explains. 'The hospital nutritionist put me on an exercise programme and a low-calorie diet. I started walking for 20 minutes a few times a week, and I began eating several mini-meals throughout the day, instead of the all-day meal I used to eat. My husband was a great support – he measured all my food and created my menus. He helped me learn about portion sizes. I was surprised to learn, for instance, that a piece of cheese as long as the distance from the tip of your index finger to your first knuckle constitutes one serving, and there are 100 calories in that serving.

'After I got out of hospital, I continued eating four or five mini-meals throughout the day. I have breakfast, lunch, dinner and a night-time snack of a rice cake or some sugar-free jelly, and occasionally I have a mid-morning snack as well.

'I eat smaller portions and make better food choices. I used to eat eggs and bacon for breakfast, but now I eat half a grapefruit, a serving of porridge with skimmed milk, half a bagel and, of course, coffee. I haven't eliminated any foods from my diet, except sweets because of my diabetes. I've just learned to recognize what serving sizes are, and I apply that knowledge to whatever I eat.

'I have also kept up with my exercise plan, and now I walk 4 to 5.5 km (2½ to 3½ miles) five times a week. Walking coupled with my new mini-meal habits has helped me maintain my weight at 57 kg (9 st) for the past three years. And it has done wonders for my diabetes!'

Choose no-risk foods. As you adapt, choose low-calorie foods. Reach for the fat-free milk, apples and air-popped popcorn, or a sweet potato and a mixed green salad dressed with lemon juice or balsamic vinegar. (Say no thanks to the Caesar salad and chips.)

Go to pieces. Mini-meals will be more satisfying if you eat them in small bites. So instead of one big rice cake, have a few of the bite-size variety. Or cut a biscuit into pieces and eat the pieces individually.

Don't tempt yourself. If you know that you have no resistance to certain foods – biscuits, for example – stay away from them. If you don't, you'll probably end up eating well beyond fullness. Choose mini-meal foods that you know you can control, says Donna Weihofen, a nutritionist.

Watch out for fat-free. Most of the new packaged fat-free foods won't fill you up for long. Also, many fat-free foods have added sugar to make up for the loss of fat. Look at the total calories, not just the fat – many of these foods are only 20 or so calories lower than the full-fat version! (And trust us – if you've ever walked for half an hour on a treadmill, only to discover at the end that you've burned a total of 150 calories, a 20-calorie drop isn't *nearly* low enough!)

Be a Time Machine

You might be afraid that eating six meals a day would really cut into your time. But remember – these are mini-meals, not formal dinners. Eating mini-meals doesn't have to be time-consuming, according to Natalie Payne, a nutritionist. Here are some time-saving strategies.

Take mini-meals on the road. Keep a snack stash in your car, carry snacks in your handbag when you go shopping, and stock your briefcase when you fly. Good portables include small boxes of raisins, mini-boxes of cereal, cartons of vegetable juice and wholewheat crackers. (This practice has another benefit: if you find yourself ravenous on the road or at the shopping centre or airport, you won't be tempted to grab the closest high-calorie fast-food!)

Switch meals. Consider some easy-to-prepare, easy-to-eat (but somewhat unusual) choices for your meals. Make a turkey sandwich in the evening, for example, and put it in the fridge. Then grab it on your way out the door in the morning and eat it for breakfast on your way to work.

Keep it cold. If you don't have access to a refrigerator where you work, freeze a carton of juice overnight and put it in the bottom of your lunch box the following day. The frozen juice will keep easy-to-eat items such as yoghurt and cheese cold.

Stash some safe bets. At work, keep a desk drawer stocked with tinned fruit (in water or fruit juice), dried fruit, low-fat crackers and other non-perishable convenience foods. (And don't forget a tin opener.)

Slice at night. When cutting up carrots and other raw vegetables for dinner, don't forget to slice some extras to take along and munch the next day at work.

Dinner – Don't Overdo It

Dinner can be the toughest time to eat a mini-meal. If you go out to eat, you're served too much food. If you eat at home, you might linger at the table with the family and eat more than you planned. Yet calories consumed at night are most likely to pack on the weight, as your metabolism actually slows while you sleep.

Here are some of nutritionists Anne Dubner and Michele Harvey's most effective ideas for downsizing your meals at dinner time and stopping yourself from overeating.

Have a starter. Have a snack ready in the fridge for when you walk in the door after work. After you've eaten your starter, change into comfortable clothes, take a shower or do whatever else you do to ready yourself for an evening meal with your family. Then you can spend as much time at the dinner table as you like, but you won't overeat because you won't be as hungry.

Don't stay on course. Switch back and forth between courses by alternating bites of your main dish (chicken or pasta, for example) with a bite of salad. If you do that, you won't finish eating before the rest of your family does.

Fill 'er up. Before ordering dinner in a restaurant, drink a big glass of water to quell your appetite. Then take a sip of water after every bite so that you'll eat more slowly.

Leave the bread. Ask the waiter not to serve bread. Or take one wholegrain roll and send the basket back.

DROP THE DIET AND START LOSING WEIGHT

For 20 years, Ann has been a chronic yo-yo dieter – up 5 kg (11 lb), down 2, up 2, down 5. Either she's dieting to starvation by existing on raw vegetables and tinned tuna or eating all the wrong things. For Ann, there is no in-between. Lately, though, she seems to have more 'eating days' than 'diet days', and her weight just keeps going up. What's happened to her willpower?

The reality is that Ann's new weight problem may have nothing to do with willpower. As we've seen, as a woman approaches menopause, her metabolism slows and she may gain weight even when eating and exercising the same way she always did. And in Ann's case, her constant dieting may have made her situation even worse. After so many years of dieting, Ann's body is probably tired from all the bouncing up and down on the scales. And like all yo-yo dieters, she has probably set unrealistic goals. When she keeps falling short of meeting them, she loses her desire to even try to fight her weight gain. For women like her, a sensible weight loss of only a pound a week is viewed as failure. Like many yo-yo dieters, she eats out of frustration for failing and promises to start all over again tomorrow.

It's going to be difficult for Ann to reclaim her willpower as it's been years since she's eaten sensibly. But she can do it if she changes her habits. First, she needs to set realistic weight-loss goals. She needs to realize that the only way she'll achieve long-term success is through gradual steps. If she doesn't lose weight right away, she shouldn't consider herself a failure.

Second, she needs to believe that all foods are allowed; otherwise, the foods she deprives herself of on her 'diet days' are exactly the foods she'll want on her 'eating days'. Most important, she needs to get on a regular eating plan with three small meals a day, spaced fairly evenly, and enough snacks in between to keep her from bingeing later on. Once Ann stops playing yo-yo with her eating habits, her weight is bound to settle down, too.

Request less. Ask the waiter for a smaller portion. You could request a meal that's half the usual size, for example.

Don't order your main course right away. When eating out, have a small bowl of non–creamy soup like minestrone or a small salad before making a decision on your main course. That way, you won't be as hungry and you'll order a smaller meal.

Or don't order it at all. Instead of ordering a main course, order a starter.

Start low, end high. Eat your vegetables first, then the starches, such as potatoes and bread. Leave the highest-calorie and fattiest items, like meat, for last. That way you'll fill up on the lowest-calorie items and feel too full to finish the high-calorie foods.

Take it home. Before the waiter brings the meal, ask for a doggie bag. When he brings the dinner, immediately divide your food, putting half in the take-away container and leaving the rest on your plate. Or ask the waiter to do it for you. Store the take-away container under your chair so you won't be tempted to nibble from it.

Don't worry about detours. Every once in a while – at Christmas, for example – you'll stuff yourself. Don't feel guilty. 'You are not going to get lost when you take a detour, as long as you don't keep slapping yourself across the face,' says Michele Harvey. You will get lost, however, if you continually berate yourself, she says, because then you'll feel so bad about yourself that you'll keep eating.

More Tricks for Keeping the 'Mini' in Mini-meals

It's obvious that if you're eating mini-meals but you don't downsize each meal, you won't lose weight. But how can you keep the portions from creeping up on you? Here are some top-notch tips from Edith Howard Hogan, a nutrition counsellor specializing in women's health and a spokesperson for the American Dietetic Association.

- **Choose 'one-fisted' snacks.** A piece of fresh fruit, a miniature box of raisins, a pot of yoghurt, a little box of cereal, a snack-sized carton of fruit juice, or a one-portion sized tin of tuna automatically limits your portions.

- **Shrink your sweets.** Bite-sized chocolate bars, pre-sliced cakes or mini bagels will give you the taste you love with portion control. Just be sure to say no to seconds.

- **Downsize your dishes.** Use a salad plate instead of a dinner plate for meals, a cup instead of a bowl for soup and a juice glass

BALANCE YOUR PORTIONS

Here's another trick for minimizing menopausal weight gain. Select the right balance of foods on your plate, says Jackie Newgent, an instructor at a prestigious cooking school. Jackie's message is slice starches, dice fat, value vegetables!

Menopause slows your metabolic rate. To compensate, one of your best moves is to limit fat consumption. 'But the downside of cutting too much fat is that it leaves you hungry,' says Jackie. Many people then make the mistake of taking gluttonous helpings of carbohydrates instead. Then they find to their horror that their waistlines keep expanding.

The key to success, according to Jackie, is to practise just as much portion control with breads and pastas as with cheese and meat portions. If you're hungry, load up on veggies and pulses.

'It's just a matter of balance,' Jackie says. 'Remember that less fat, fewer starches, and more vegetables will help you maintain your premenopausal waistline and ease the burden on your postmenopausal heart.'

This Confetti Veggie Couscous is a quick and delicious example of a balanced one-dish meal.

---

instead of a tumbler for drinks (unless it's water, which you want to load up on).

- **Take control.** Finally, remember these wise words from Edith: 'When your eating is under control, everything else feels more in control, too. Instead of eating for comfort and making everything worse, eat for health and energy to support positive change.'

Eating for an Easier Menopause

Mini-meals will help you keep mid-life weight gain under control, but they won't do much to minimize menopause's more unpleasant symptoms (hot flushes come to mind). Fortunately, there's plenty you can do to help

Confetti Veggie Couscous

1	tablespoon extra-virgin olive oil
3	large cloves garlic, crushed
600 ml (1 pint)	vegetable stock
150 g (5 oz)	chopped red peppers
150 g (5 oz)	chopped courgettes
90 g (3 oz)	grated carrot
300 g (10½ oz)	wholewheat couscous
2 tablespoons	chopped fresh oregano, basil, parsley, or a mixture
	Salt to taste
	Lemon juice

Add the oil to a large saucepan over medium heat. Add the garlic and cook for about 1 minute, being careful not to brown the garlic. Add the stock, peppers, courgettes and carrot. Bring just to a boil over high heat. Stir in the couscous and herbs. Cover and immediately remove from the heat. Let sit for 5 minutes. Fluff with a fork and add salt. Serve immediately or chilled with a squirt of fresh lemon juice.

MAKES 6 SERVINGS

yourself have an easier menopause just by making the right food choices. We'll give you specific disease-fighting foods in the sections on the big menopausal diseases – cancer (page 43), osteoporosis (page 46), and heart disease (page 50) – that follow. But first, we'd like to present a few foods and drinks that we think *all* menopausal women should include in their diets for reduction of menopausal symptoms, overall well-being and preventive care. And there are a few foods and drinks that you should avoid. Here are our top recommendations.

Avoid 'Flush' Foods

Tea, coffee and other hot or spicy foods and drinks can provoke the sweaty spells we all dread. During menopause, your body struggles to control its internal thermostat. All too often, it fails. Toss in caffeine, with its stimulating effects, and things get worse. Serve it up hot, and if you're prone to hot flushes, you'd better head for the deep freeze.

'I tell my patients that hot coffee and hot tea are no-nos if they want to minimize hot flushes,' says Mary Jane Minkin, clinical professor of obstetrics and gynaecology at Yale University School of Medicine and co-author of *What Every Woman Needs to Know About Menopause*. Hot drinks add warmth to your body, and this burst of heat can overload your erratic temperature mechanisms. Caffeine also relaxes your capillaries and allows more blood and heat to reach your skin, creating the unwelcome flush. Alcohol has a similar warming effect.

Spicy foods can also superstimulate more than just your tongue. Limit your intake of whole peppercorns, crushed red pepper and even freshly ground pepper, says Dr Minkin. Steer clear of chillis in Mexican, Thai, Indian and Chinese foods. Remember that the smaller the chilli, the hotter it will usually be.

Don't Forget Fibre!

In terms of warding off diseases that often strike at mid-life, fibre may be the most important dietary supplement ever. There's evidence that a high-fibre diet may help protect against breast cancer. It can also help to lower blood cholesterol, stabilize blood sugar in women with diabetes, and prevent intestinal ills – constipation, diarrhoea, haemorrhoids, diverticulosis, even colon cancer.

As the indigestible part of plants, fibre isn't absorbed by the body. It travels pretty much intact from the stomach to the intestines. There it soaks up water like a sponge, softening and bulking up the stool so it moves through the intestine quickly and efficiently. This not only alleviates many bowel disturbances; it also prevents harmful, cancer-causing substances from camping out and getting a stronghold. Fibre's amazing cholesterol-lowering effect is achieved in the same process. While absorbing water in the intestines, fibre also sucks up bile, a fluid secreted by the liver that aids digestion. To make more bile, the liver pilfers cholesterol from the bloodstream, resulting in lower blood cholesterol.

HOW TO EAT MORE FIBRE

Want to make sure you're getting plenty of lifesaving fibre? Eat your cereal. Not surprisingly, some breakfast cereals top the charts for fibre content. Just one 50-g serving of Kellogg's All-Bran packs a whopping 13.5 g. One 50-g serving of Kellogg's Bran Flakes contains 7.5 g. A 50-g serving of Kellogg's Sultana Bran has 6 g. Here are a dozen more sources of fibre that can help you get closer to meeting your daily needs.

- Butter beans, 100 g (3½ oz): 4.6 g
- Dried figs, 100 g (3½ oz): 7.5 g
- Dried apricots, 100 g (3½ oz): 6.3 g
- Kidney beans, 100 g (3½ oz): 6.7 g
- Artichoke, one medium: 6.5 g
- Lentils, 100 g (3½ oz): 3.8 g
- Potato with skin, one baked: 4.8 g
- Raspberries, 100 g (3½ oz): 2.5 g
- Chick peas, 100 g (3½ oz): 4.3 g
- Apple with peel, one medium: 3.7 g
- Blackberries, 100 g (3½ oz): 3.1 g
- Sweet potato, baked, one medium: 3.4 g

If that's not enough to win you over, fibre has been called the most powerful weight-loss aid in the world. That's because high–fibre foods make you feel full on fewer calories. And when you're fighting off 'menopause middle', that's really good news.

Getting Enough

In spite of its many benefits, few women get the recommended 20 to 40 grams of fibre per day – the amount studies suggest for blanket health protection. Most of us get half that amount or less. Yet fibre is extremely easy to add to your diet. Just incorporate fruit, vegetables, pulses (beans and peas) and whole grains such as oats and whole wheat. Or, for an extra boost, supplement your meals with a granulated fibre product such as wheat bran, or psyllium. But don't rely solely on fibre supplements to meet your recommended daily requirements. You'll miss out on the disease-fighting vitamins and minerals that are available only in food.

Don't forget to drink lots of water, at least eight 240-ml (8-fl oz) glasses a day, while eating a high-fibre diet and/or taking fibre supplements. If you run dry, you risk becoming constipated or experiencing other unpleasant intestinal disturbances such as wind (already a common problem during the menopause) or a more serious complication such as a bowel obstruction.

The Menopause Superfood: Soya

Soya's extraordinary potential to relieve hot flushes and other meno-pausal symptoms and reduce cholesterol has made it *the* superfood for menopausal women. (For more on soya's role in fighting high cholesterol, see 'Enjoy Soya's Flour Power' on page 35.) Soya may also fight breast cancer, protect against colon cancer and endometrial cancer, and prevent strokes – among other life-extending benefits.

'There almost isn't a disease that soya can't help in some way,' says Dr John Glaspy, who is studying soya's protective effect against breast cancer.

The 'magic' ingredients responsible for soya's healing prowess? Isoflavones – specifically genistein and daidzein – oestrogen-like com-pounds abundant in soya beans. Soya is 'the' life extension food. Doctors and scientists add soya to their diets, and advise women to do the same.

One of the richest sources of isoflavones (about 25 mg per 100 g) is tofu – sponge-like blocks of soya bean curd sold in supermarkets. But if you're like many women, you know your family will never, ever eat it. (And you're not too fond of it yourself.) It's soft, mushy and bland.

Chinese, Vietnamese and Thai cuisines work wonders with tofu, changing the texture so it's chewy or crispy and adding a variety of robust, mouthwatering flavours. We suggest that you try a few tofu (often listed as 'bean curd' in Chinese restaurants) dishes when you're eating out and see if your opinion of tofu improves.

Still can't face tofu, or just want to get the benefits of soya more often than the occasional Chinese take-away? No problem. Here's a list of 15 *other* tasty ways to work soya into your diet without eating tofu, starting with those with the highest isoflavone content per serving. (Isoflavone

BE SOYA SAVVY

Soya is loaded with oestrogen-like plant substances, which in moderation may help replace your body's subsiding hormone reserves. Women in Japan and China eat lots of soya foods. These women also don't need hormone replacement therapy (HRT) since they have few menopausal symptoms, not to mention low rates of breast cancer. Better yet, research suggests that plant hormones in soya called isoflavones are responsible for building bone, thus lowering the risk for osteoporosis, which normally soars in menopausal years. Studies show that another plant hormone in soya, genistein, shows promise in fighting cancerous tumours.

Can eating soya help you to avoid menopausal problems as it does for your sisters living in the Far East? The medical community is not sure. Researchers have a number of misgivings and unanswered questions about this ancient Asian wonder.

'The truth is, the Asian women who avoid symptoms have been eating soya all of their lives and may be benefiting from other factors in their diets or lifestyle,' says Dr Walter Willett, professor of epidemiology and nutrition and chairperson of the department of nutrition at the Harvard School of Public Health. In fact, some studies suggest that adding excessive doses of plant oestrogens, like those found in soya products, to your diet later in life may actually *increase* your cancer risk.

So what should you do about this promising but perplexing food? Dr Willett recommends incorporating soya into your diet, within limits. One or two servings of soya foods daily may be enough to give your oestrogen a little lift, especially if you forgo HRT (women on hormone replacement therapy shouldn't need any help). Try calcium-fortified sweetened soya milk on your cereal. Snack on roasted soya nuts from the healthfood shop. Marinate sliced tofu and portobello mushrooms, then grill and throw the mixture into a pitta pocket or into pasta.

content varies from product to product.) Many are found in supermarkets; others, in healthfood shops or by mail order.

- Textured vegetable protein – 62 milligrams of isoflavones per 15 g (½ oz) of dry granules. Use as a meat substitute in chilli, spaghetti bolognese and shepherd's pie

- Soya shakes – 52 to 57 milligrams of isoflavones (smooth, creamy drinks from milk and fat-free ice cream)

- Soya protein bars – 49 milligrams of isoflavones per bar (available in a number of different flavours)

- Tinned soya beans – 41 milligrams of isoflavones per 90 g (3 oz) (chestnutty and creamy; they work well in soups and chilli)

- Tempeh – 36 milligrams of isoflavones per 90 g (3 oz) (sold in cakes, then marinated, sliced and fried)

- Soya milk – 30 milligrams of isoflavones per 240 ml (8 fl oz) (a slightly beany liquid best used in shakes, puddings and hot chocolate, though vanilla soya milk poured over cereal is tasty)

- Roasted soya nuts – 30 milligrams of isoflavones per 3 tablespoons (look like tiny peanuts – delicious as a snack)

- Soya desserts – 30 milligrams of isoflavones per 90 g (3 oz)

- Miso – 29 milligrams of isoflavones per 75 g (2½ oz) (a flavouring for soups and stews; tastes a little like teriyaki)

- Soya cheese – 9 milligrams of isoflavones per 30 g (1 oz) (used in cooking as a non-dairy stand-in for the real thing. If you don't like one soya cheese, try a different brand. Tastes and textures vary.)

- Soya burgers – 8 milligrams of isoflavones per burger (an easy-to-digest substitute for beef, it tastes a little like bean dip with vegetables)

- Soya flour – 8 milligrams of isoflavones per tablespoon (replace one-quarter to one-third of the flour in recipes for cakes and other baked goods – you'll never taste the difference)

- Soya ice cream – 5 milligrams of isoflavones per 75 g (2½ oz)

Experts recommend that you get 30 to 50 milligrams of isoflavones a day – easy with so much variety.

> # PLEASE READ THE LABELS!
>
> Not every soya product automatically supplies isoflavones. Avoid 'soya protein concentrate' – most of the isoflavones may have been processed out. Instead, look for 'isolated soya protein', 'soya protein isolate', or 'textured soya protein' on the label. (If you're unsure, write to or call the manufacturer.) Roasted soya butter has only 1 milligram of isoflavone per serving. And don't count on soy sauce or soya bean oil – they contain *no* isoflavones.

Helpful Hints

Plain soya milk is off-white and beany tasting. Look for chocolate, vanilla or other flavours. Or stir in some cocoa powder, coffee, almond extract or whatever strikes your fancy. For example, heat 240 ml (8 fl oz) of soya milk in the microwave for one minute, add a little instant coffee or drinking chocolate powder, and you have a healthy and delicious latte or hot chocolate.

Go against the Grain

Westerners are virtually addicted to white flour, white rice and white sugar. Perhaps refined foods may look and feel lighter. But in reality, it's the darker, whole grains that can keep *you* lighter – and keep you alive longer.

When the diets of 34,000 women aged 55 to 69 were analysed by researchers at the University of Minnesota, those who had diets high in whole grains were 40 per cent more likely to live longer. Women who ate at least one daily serving of whole grains had a substantially lower risk of cancer, cardiovascular disease, diabetes and other diseases than women who ate almost no whole grains. And there's more good news: the whole grain eaters were significantly slimmer than the fans of refined foods.

'Women who eat more fibre usually weigh less, making it a welcome ally in the battle against menopausal weight gain and heart disease. That may be because high-fibre foods tend to be low in calories, yet bulky and filling, and they take longer to digest than processed foods,' says Dr Christine Rosenbloom, an associate professor of nutrition.

Although the processed food industry so often removes stay-slim fibre from common foods, make the effort to get the right grain. When the germ and hulls are removed to make white flour and white rice, for instance, they lose fibre, along with precious nutrients. Whole grains, on the other hand, tend to be more satisfying because of their fuller, more satisfying flavours as well as the chewier textures that you can really sink your teeth into.

Most women eat 12 to 14 grams of fibre daily. But actually, you need to eat twice that amount, particularly as you go through menopause, says Dr Rosenbloom. A great habit to increase fibre is to do your own baking with whole flours and oat bran, and base lots of meals around brown rice and wild rice, bulgur wheat and buckwheat (kasha).

When you do buy processed foods, let the numbers talk. A 'high-fibre' food supplies 6 or more grams per 100 g serving, while a food labelled as 'a source of fibre' provides at least 3 grams per 100 g serving. Look for multigrain or wholegrain cereals and savoury biscuits, and switch to wholewheat pasta, pitta bread and tortillas. For a bigger fibre boost, mash up bran cereal and use it as a topping for casseroles, vegetables, fruit, even frozen yoghurt. And don't forget popcorn – it's truly a fibre-friendly snack.

Wheatgerm: Treat This Germ like a Gem

Wheatgerm is packed with so many nutrients that many researchers consider it the ultimate health food for menopausal women. It's a concentrated source of vitamin E and folate, both of which have been shown to protect against heart disease, says Densie Webb, a nutritionist. 'It's also packed with manganese, magnesium, phosphorus and potassium – trace minerals recently shown to be critical for strong bones.'

Wheatgerm is a part of the wheat kernel, which, along with the fibrous bran coating, gets processed out to make white flour, so most women don't get very much of it. But you can add it back into your diet in a variety of ways. When you're baking cakes or breads, substitute about 75 g (2½ oz) of flour with wheatgerm. In biscuits, go up to 150 g (5 oz). You can also swirl it into smoothies or yoghurt, or sprinkle it on cold cereal and salads.

At room temperature, wheatgerm spoils quickly, so refrigerate it in a tightly sealed container. That way, it will stay fresh for up to nine months, says Dr Webb.

Water Down Symptoms

Being even a little dehydrated can trigger a range of menopause aggravations. So drink up.

Staying well-hydrated is vital for cooling down those hot flushes and fending off constipation, irritability, insomnia and other symptoms of menopause.

Getting enough water also can help you feel more energetic and can even diminish skin dryness.

Here are a few solid ways to avoid dehydration and to minimize menopausal symptoms.

- Drink six to eight 240-ml (8-fl oz) glasses of water daily. If you're active, especially in hot and humid weather, drink more.

- Cool water is absorbed more quickly into your body than warm water. So chill your water bottle in a freezer for a few minutes before you head out to the golf course or tennis court. Your water is also more apt to stay cold until the end of your game.

- Tap water is fine, but if you prefer the flavour or carbonation of bottled water, that works just as well. Do whatever it takes to keep your tank full.

- Limit your consumption of cola, coffee and other caffeinated drinks as they are diuretics, which move water out of your body.

- Think you're hungry? Have a glass of water first. Thirst often masquerades as hunger.

Cutting Your Cancer Risk

As if the thought of cancer weren't already frightening enough, the risks of certain kinds of cancer, including breast cancer and endometrial cancer, rise after menopause. (See 'Colour Your Life with Cancer Protection' below for more on breast cancer risks.) If you choose to combat menopausal symptoms with hormone replacement therapy (HRT), new studies show that your risk of developing breast cancer can rise even higher.

So it's a smart move for all of us, as we enter menopause, to start doing everything we comfortably can to reduce our cancer risks. And one of the easiest things we can do is to modify our diets. Even small changes – such as adding more of the fruit and vegetables we all know we *should* be eating anyway – can make a big difference. Read on for tasty ways to add cancer-fighting foods and flavourings to your daily meals.

Colour Your Life with Cancer Protection

Many postmenopausal women fear breast cancer – and with good reason. The older you get, the higher your risk of this dreaded diagnosis. One out of eight women experience breast cancer by the age of 80. But there's something that can protect you, and fortunately, it's in your garden, says Cyndi Thomson, a diet and breast cancer researcher at the University of Arizona.

Eat a minimum of seven servings of fruit and vegetables daily in all hues of the rainbow, she suggests. That's because carotenoids, the plant chemicals that create bright colours in fruit and vegetables, may help prevent cancer. Make it a habit to dine on blueberries, grapes, raisins or sultanas, plums, mango, dark green lettuce, spinach, kale, carrots, strawberries, tomatoes, beets and red, green, orange and yellow peppers.

Try a new fruit or vegetable each week, and learn new ways to prepare old favourites. You don't have to give up meat completely; just shift towards a more colourful, plant-based diet. A good tool for expanding your produce menu is a vegetarian starter cookbook, such as *The Cranks Bible* by Nadine Abensur, *Delia's Vegetarian Collection* by Delia Smith or *Vegetarian Meals in Minutes* by Rose Elliot.

Cancer-fighting Flavourings

Non-fattening flavour enhancers will not only spice up your meals but also help you break away from eating habits that can undermine your postmenopausal health. Old family favourites may suddenly seem bland and joyless when you banish their fat-laden ingredients in order to reduce your cancer risk, lower your cholesterol and minimize your postmenopausal risk of heart disease. But there is life after cream and bacon. You can avoid dieting doldrums by flavouring food in new ways that will tempt your taste buds, protect your heart, and fight cancer, too.

Here's how:

- Start by replacing butter with extra-virgin olive oil. The flavour is robust, so you don't need much. And for weight control, think

---

HEALTHY, HEARTY PASTA

The next time you think 'spaghetti', skip the meatballs and, instead, try this Chickpea Pasta Sauce from Jackie Newgent, cooking instructor at a prestigious cooking school.

Chickpea Pasta Sauce

> 1   tablespoon extra-virgin olive oil
> 1   large onion, thinly sliced
> 2–3   cloves garlic, crushed
> 1   tin (400 g or 14 oz) chickpeas
> 1   tin (400 g or 14 oz) chopped tomatoes, with juice
> 1   tablespoon chopped or crushed fresh rosemary
>   Salt and freshly ground pepper
>   Hot-pepper sauce
> 2   tablespoons freshly grated Parmesan cheese (optional)

Heat the oil in a large saucepan over medium heat. Cover the pan with a tight-fitting lid and 'sweat' the onion and garlic by allowing them to soften and slowly release their own water without browning. If they begin to brown, reduce the heat.

In a blender, purée half the chickpeas. Add a little water to thin the mixture if necessary. Stir the puréed chickpeas, whole chickpeas, tomatoes (with juice), and rosemary into the onion-garlic mixture. Simmer, uncovered, stirring occasionally for about 20 minutes, or until the sauce thickens.

Season with salt and pepper and the hot-pepper sauce. Stir in the Parmesan, if using. Serve over your favourite pasta or couscous or use as a sauce for baked or grilled chicken.

Makes 8 servings

teaspoons, not tablespoons. Olive oil supplies a more heart-healthy kind of fat, but it's still high in calories.

• Cook with plenty of onions and fresh garlic, too. They're rich in organosulphides, compounds that create their characteristic 'fragrances' and protect against heart disease and cancer. For best flavour and least fat, learn to 'sweat' your vegetables (you sweat an onion, for example, by allowing it to soften and slowly release its own water, without browning it).

• Experiment with different herbs. Rosemary in particular is good. Its pine fragrance entices you to indulge in dishes even if they lack the familiar smack of saturated fat. Rosemary is also packed with carnosol, an antioxidant that may prevent cancer.

• One last trick: replacing minced beef with beans will eliminate the saturated fat and load you up on antioxidants that can defend cells against cancer-causing agent.

Give Your Bones a Break from Osteoporosis

We've all got enough to do without worrying about broken bones. But osteoporosis is one of the major diseases women face after the menopause, and along with it comes the spectre of dowager's humps and broken hips. Some 40 per cent of women in the UK suffer an osteoporosis-induced fracture in their lifetime. In Australia, the US and New Zealand, one in two women over the age of 60 will suffer a fracture due to osteoporosis. Decades of chronic pain and disfigurement can follow all-too-common vertebral compression fractures. If the injury is to the hip, a woman's golden years are likely to be blackened by permanent disability or premature death. Roughly one-quarter of the people who survive hip fractures require long-term care.

Needless to say, it's imperative to take this insidious disease seriously, particularly when oestrogen decline at menopause increases its likelihood. So start protecting your bones now with weight-bearing exercises (for more on these, see Chapter 3, 'The Menopause Exercise Plan') and bone-strengthening foods and supplements.

Catch Up with Calcium

Calcium helps to slow bone loss after the menopause. But to get enough each day, you must think beyond the obvious. When the menopause occurs, a woman can begin losing up to 7 per cent of her bone mass annually. Over time, that loss can lead to osteoporosis, the bone-thinning disease known as the silent crippler of women.

The current recommendation for calcium intake is 700 mg for women aged 19–50 years. However, the National Osteoporosis Society recommends higher intakes of up to 1500 mg per day for women over 45. The recommended daily requirement for calcium is found in just over a pint of semi-skimmed milk, 100 g of cheddar cheese or 400 g of natural yoghurt. In Australia, the NHMRC recommends 800 mg per day for women between the ages of 19 and 54, and 1000 mg for women after the menopause. These figures are the same in New Zealand and South Africa. To get an optimum daily dose, you're probably going to have to make a few changes in your diet.

Here are just a few ways to enhance your calcium intake.

- Sprinkle 30 g (1 oz) of grated low-fat cheese on your salad, and you get another 200 milligrams of calcium.
- Top 100 g (3½ oz) of steamed broccoli with a tablespoon of sesame seeds, and get a vegetarian bonanza worth 82 milligrams of calcium.
- Scatter 2 tablespoons of sliced almonds on your green beans and get a 50-milligram calcium bonus.
- Eat more beans. Most contain between 50 and 130 milligrams of calcium per 100 g (3½ oz).

Get Hip to Vitamin K

If you're trying to avoid fractures caused by menopause-related bone loss, maybe you're eating plenty of dairy foods already. But a lesser-known security for your skeleton is to increase your vitamin K intake.

Research shows that middle-aged women who get the most vitamin K from food have the lowest rates of hip fractures.

'Green vegetables are the best source of vitamin K, which activates osteocalcin, a protein that makes your bones stronger,' says Liz Ward, a nutritionist and co-author of *Super Nutrition after 50*. Just one brussels sprout or 60 g (2 oz) of broccoli, spring greens, cabbage, spinach or kale will do it. For variety, try 90 g (3 oz) of cooked asparagus or green beans or 60 g (2 oz) of cauliflower. Vitamin K is also found in soya bean oil and egg yolks.

Yell for Yoghurt

Want a supercharged source of calcium to strengthen your menopausal bones? Put yoghurt at the top of your shopping list. Yoghurt is a plain and simple skeleton helper. Plain yoghurt packs a whopping 400 milligrams of calcium per 200 g (7 oz), and it's more readily digested than milk, says JoAnn Hattner, a nutrition counsellor.

In fact, as we age and head towards menopause, many of us lose the ability to break down lactose, the sugar in milk, and end up with bloating, cramping or diarrhoea. Many women who can't handle milk, however, do just fine with yoghurt. That's because, in the yoghurt-making process, friendly bacteria digest a lot of the lactose for us.

Also, with age, many women experience mild gastrointestinal symptoms. 'Live and active cultures in yoghurt keep your intestinal tract healthier,' says JoAnn. And that's in contrast to the problems some women have with calcium supplements. 'Among the women I counsel, some become constipated from calcium carbonate supplements, while others develop loose stools from calcium supplements that contain magnesium. I tell them they'll do better with low-fat or fat-free yoghurt.'

JoAnn shares another bone-friendly tip: 'In its natural state, plain yoghurt is higher in calcium than sweetened varieties. You can sweeten it yourself with honey and get a bonus because honey seems to fight infection.'

You can use yoghurt as a condiment by dolloping it on top of soups and mixing it with grated lime peel as an accompaniment for fruit. Or try this simple, luscious yoghurt-based dip for vegetables.

Creamy Mustard Dip

Use as a dip for fresh vegetables or dried tomatoes.

200 g (7 oz)	low-fat cottage cheese
100 g (3½ oz)	low-fat plain yoghurt
2 tablespoons	Dijon mustard
1	teaspoon chopped fresh thyme
2	teaspoons minced shallots
1	teaspoon chopped fresh dill or ¼ teaspoon dried
½	teaspoon lemon juice

In a food processor or blender, whip the cottage cheese until smooth. Add the yoghurt, mustard, thyme, shallots, dill and lemon juice. Stir until blended.

Say 'Cheese!' for a Healthy Smile

When we think of postmenopausal bone loss, we tend to think of hip fractures and spinal compression. But there's another set of critical bones that need protection: your skull and jawbone. Calcium loss in the jaws can lead to loose (and ultimately lost) teeth. The teeth themselves can suffer from calcium loss.

After menopause, your gums are also more vulnerable to decay. That's because the loss of oestrogen that occurs during menopause affects all the cells in your body, including the gum tissue surrounding your teeth. As your gums recede, tooth roots, which are not protected by hard enamel, become exposed to dental-caries-causing bacteria. And to make matters worse, baked, starchy foods such as pastries, biscuits and cakes stick between your teeth, providing the bacteria and the acidic conditions that rot teeth. Dry mouth, another menopause symptom and a side-effect of some medications, can also lead to gum disease.

For past generations, the answer to tooth loss was dentures, something that seemed as inevitable as reading glasses. But women today would like to keep their own teeth, thank you. And because of better at-home dental care and routine dental cleanings, we have a better chance of doing so than our mothers and grandmothers.

Our food choices can also help in the fight to keep our teeth. Just chomping on a piece or two of cheese, such as Swiss, Cheddar or Red Leicester, every day may actually protect against decay, says Mary P. Faine, associate professor of nutrition at the University of Washington. Dairy products, and cheese in particular, contain a protein that prevents plaque from sticking to teeth, she says.

Here are other tips to smile about:

- Brushing your teeth or drinking water after snacks will help fend off decay.

- If you experience dry mouth, chew high-fibre foods, such as celery or carrots. They stimulate saliva flow, which protects your teeth.

- A glass of fat-free milk is a good saliva substitute because it won't cause decay and it helps provide the calcium you need to keep your jawbone strong and your teeth sturdy.

Heading Off Heart Disease

It wasn't so long ago that everyone thought of heart disease as a man's problem. What a shock when the news broke that it's also a major killer of women! The risk rises after menopause, so you need to act now to keep your heart healthy and your cholesterol and blood pressure low. Once again, your food choices can help you. From nuts and salmon to psyllium supplements and orange juice, here are some easy ways to pack more heart-healing punch into your meals.

Put the Crunch on Heart Disease

Pecans, almonds and other nuts can help slash your heart disease risk after menopause. It's an injustice to their other health benefits if you shun them just because they contain fat. Eating just 30 g (1 oz) daily can lower 'bad', low-density lipoprotein (LDL) cholesterol levels, slightly raise 'good', high-density lipoprotein (HDL) cholesterol levels, and lower triglyceride levels – a triple treat that protects against postmenopausal heart disease, says Kenneth I. Burke, a professor of nutrition and dietetics.

Walnuts, for example, are the best land-based source of omega-3 fatty acids, the heart-protective oil found in salmon and other cold-water fish. Pecans, just like olives, are rich in oleic acid, another cardiovascular power broker. And almonds are a bountiful source of heart-healthy natural vitamin E. Just be sure to crunch with control. Each level measuring tablespoonful of these nuts packs about 50 calories, which can lead to weight gain and, in turn, overtax your heart. So measure your portions. Sprinkle a tablespoon of toasted walnuts on your hot or cold breakfast cereal, stir a tablespoon of sliced almonds into yoghurt, or scatter 2 table-spoons of chopped pecans on a dinner salad until you've reached your daily quota.

Befriend Broccoli

Cruciferous (cabbage family) vegetables are well-established cancer fighters. Now comes word that broccoli is also a potent ally in your fight against postmenopausal heart disease.

Like apples and onions, broccoli is a good source of flavonoids, a group of antioxidant compounds that scavenge free radicals before they can oxidize low-density lipoprotein (LDL) cholesterol. If oxidized, this bad cholesterol can stick onto your artery walls, increasing your heart attack risk.

Researchers at the University of Minnesota hailed broccoli after they analysed the eating habits of 34,000 postmenopausal women. After 10 years, those women who had eaten the most flavonoid-laden foods had a 32 per cent lower risk of dying from heart disease than those who had eaten the least of this nutrient. Of all the beneficial foods studied, broc-coli demonstrated the most promise.

'This is the only study done exclusively on postmenopausal women that looked at flavonoids,' explains Laura Yochum, a senior health care analyst, who was the study's lead researcher. 'It suggests that getting plenty of foods rich in flavonoids, especially broccoli, can lower the heart disease risks that escalate after menopause.'

Cooked broccoli is also a good source of heart-friendly fibre and folate, as well as vitamins A, C and E. To get the most nutritional benefit, buy broccoli that is bright emerald green with small, tightly closed flower buds, she says.

Get Hooked on Deep-sea Fish

Eating certain fish can help keep your arteries clear and lower your risk of heart problems as you go through the menopause. As the menopause kicks in and your oestrogen levels tumble, your risk of heart disease shoots up. But adding fish such as salmon, turbot, haddock and cod to your menu two or three times a week can help keep your cardiovascular system healthy.

That's because these deep-water ocean fish have developed a kind of body fat – called omega-3 – that stays pliable no matter how low the temperature goes. When you eat these omega-3s, they become part of your own cell membranes, which in turn become more supple. That means the walls of your arteries are more flexible and the platelets in your blood are more slippery, a combination that can lower your risk of blood clots. (A

TAKE IRON INTAKE TO HEART

After the menopause, your body's iron requirements change. You'll need to adjust your intake to protect your heart – and your overall health.

As long as you were having regular menstrual periods, you lost precious iron, critical for carrying oxygen for energy. That's why you always needed more iron than your mate (12–15 milligrams daily to his 10 milligrams) to avoid iron deficiency anaemia. But after menopause, your iron needs drop to about 8 milligrams daily.

You still need this mineral, but you must make your intake more moderate, insists Kathleen Zelman, a spokesperson for the American Dietetic Association. Some researchers suspect that excess iron can damage the heart and other cells in the body.

To get the right age-adjusted iron dose, take a 50+ formula daily multivitamin that contains 4 milligrams of iron, she suggests. Get your remaining daily iron needs from food.

Iron from lean meat, chicken and fish is absorbed better than the iron from plant sources, such as beans, bread, fruit and vegetables. Animal protein also increases the absorption of iron from those plant sources. So add 30–60 g (1–2 oz) of chicken to your beans, have a slice of lean meat with your potatoes, or have a bit of fish with your pasta. 'You'll get all the iron you need without overdoing it,' says Kathleen.

blood clot that gets stuck in the artery that supplies blood to your heart is what typically causes a heart attack.)

Eat your fish baked, grilled, steamed, poached or even tinned. But don't fry it – that only adds heart-clogging saturated fat to your meal. When you're eating out, order grilled salmon, have anchovies on your Caesar salad or go for a tuna sandwich.

Take Psyllium with Supper

Throughout your childbearing years, oestrogen keeps cholesterol under control, providing natural protection against heart disease. But with menopause, oestrogen dwindles, which allows cholesterol levels – and your risk of heart disease – to soar.

Psyllium, the ground husk of the plantain plant and a well-known ingredient in laxatives, may be one of your best weapons in the battle against postmenopausal heart disease, says Dr Gail Frank, a professor of nutrition. Psyllium is loaded with soluble fibre, a gummy substance that clings to digestive secretions called bile. As this fibre passes through your digestive tract, it traps bile, which normally helps your body to absorb fat and cholesterol from food. Without bile, more cholesterol is excreted from your body.

Just a little psyllium is extremely potent: 1 tablespoon contains as much soluble fibre as *14 tablespoons* of oat bran, which is better known for its soluble fibre content. So even if you're already eating a diet low in saturated fat and cholesterol, adding 4 level teaspoons daily of ground psyllium seed husk to drinks and foods may further reduce your cholesterol load.

But beware: you can't eat psyllium by itself. It soaks up water in your digestive tract, which could cause constipation. Instead, stir it into at least 240 ml (8 fl oz) of juice or milk, or add it to biscuits, muffins or cakes in place of a few teaspoons of flour. Psyllium also works well in meat loaf because it helps soak up the juices.

Add psyllium to your diet gradually. Start with 1 teaspoon a day for about a week. Add another teaspoon each week until you reach 4 teaspoons a day. If you develop wind or bloating at some point, cut back to your previous amount. If even 1 teaspoon triggers these symptoms, stick it out for a week – your body may adjust. If it doesn't, cut back to ½ tea-spoon for a week, then gradually increase the amount as previously described.

Make sure you drink your daily requirement of at least eight large glasses of water. Getting plenty of water helps psyllium do its job. In addition, fluids will cut down on gas, bloating and other side-effects, says Dr Frank. (For more good reasons to drink lots of water, see 'Water Down Symptoms' on page 43.)

Psyllium is available at most healthfood shops. Check with your doctor before using the supplement because it may alter the absorption of some medications you are taking. And don't take psyllium if you have a bowel obstruction.

Sweeten Your Cholesterol Levels with Oranges

Help yourself to a little citrus sunshine. It's a surprising weapon in the fight against postmenopausal heart disease.

Researchers have long known that eating less saturated fat will lower levels of low-density lipoprotein (LDL), the so-called bad cholesterol. But food wasn't thought to have any effect on 'good', high-density lipoprotein (HDL) cholesterol. So Dr Elzbieta Kurowska, a nutrition researcher in the department of biochemistry at the University of Western Ontario, Canada, was surprised when a group of individuals she studied, including postmenopausal women (none on hormone replacement therapy), had a 20 per cent increase in HDL after drinking three 240-ml (8-fl oz) glasses of orange juice daily.

Oranges are packed with vitamin C, folate and other nutrients that could have a positive impact on cholesterol. But further studies will be needed to confirm Dr Kurowska's results and to pinpoint the precise mechanism.

Dr Kurowska is not advocating that you drink three glasses of orange juice a day. That's simply far too many calories for just one food, she says. Not to mention that some women in this small preliminary study developed high triglycerides, another risk factor for heart disease. Instead, she suggests that you drink one glass of orange juice daily if you are menopausal. That

SPREAD ON BENECOL'S BENEFITS

If you're tired of the battle of butter versus margarine in your low-cholesterol campaign, try Benecol on your bread. Benecol, a margarine-like spread available in most supermarkets, can help keep menopausal oestrogen loss from pushing your cholesterol sky high. More than 20 clinical studies have shown that as little as three Benecol servings daily can drop total cholesterol by 10 per cent and the 'bad', low-density lipoprotein (LDL) cholesterol by 14 per cent.

Benecol is a combination of rapeseed oil and a powerful plant compound that helps block the absorption of cholesterol in your digestive tract. Unlike some margarines, regular Benecol spread – but not the 'light' version – can be used to bake or sauté.

'It tastes good, and it actually melts,' says Dr Nadine Pazder, an outpatient dietitian. Try it on air-popped popcorn, baked potatoes, bagels, toast and cooked veggies, pasta or rice.

Although Benecol is not a drug, be sure to check with your doctor before using this product if you are taking cholesterol-lowering medication or if you are allergic to soya products.

way, you'll still probably increase your good cholesterol without causing your triglycerides to sneak upwards.

Enjoy Soya's Flour Power

While all of soya's benefits to postmenopausal women are not completely understood, it is clear that enjoying soya foods daily can lower your total cholesterol level by about 10 per cent. After the onset of menopause, a woman's total and 'bad', low-density lipoprotein (LDL) cholesterol levels are likely to rise, while her 'good', high-density lipoprotein (HDL) cholesterol levels wane, probably because of a dwindling supply of oestrogen. Soya, because of its oestrogen-like properties, may help halt that trend.

Soya flour is a concentrated source of protein, with about 37 grams per 100 g (3½ oz). It takes about 25 grams per day to get soya's cholesterol-lowering effect, says Barbara Gollman, a dietitian, nutrition educator and cookery expert. This is an amount considered safe even if you're at

DASH AWAY FROM HIGH BLOOD PRESSURE

More than half of all women over the age of 55 have high blood pressure. But dietary changes can begin to tame this 'silent killer' in as little as 14 days.

When women reach the menopause, usually in their late forties or early fifties, they are more likely than men of the same age to develop hypertension, also known as high blood pressure. Untreated, high blood pressure can lead to heart disease or stroke. But there's plenty that you can do to slash your risk of hypertension at menopause. For starters, eat less salt, lose weight and cut down on alcohol. But to really take a load off your cardiovascular system, consider adding a powerful new weapon to your hypertension-busting plan – the DASH diet.

When people tried the Dietary Approaches to Stop Hypertension (DASH) pro-gramme in research centres around the US, the results were remarkable. Research shows that shifting from a typical high-fat diet to an eating plan that's low in fat, high in fruit and vegetables and rich in low-fat dairy products can lower blood pressure as much as medication can, and in just two weeks, says Dr Lawrence J. Appel, associate professor of medicine, epidemiology and interna-tional health at the Johns Hopkins Medical Institutions.

The diet is pretty 'non-Western', as it includes about double the average con-sumption of fruit, vegetables and low-fat dairy products. But it's well worth the effort if you can get your blood pressure down without drugs, Dr Appel says.

For best results, try to stay as close as possible to the following food propor-tions used in the DASH diet. If you're taking medication for high blood pressure, don't stop without your doctor's permission.

- Grains and grain products: 7 to 8 servings daily
- Low-fat or fat-free dairy foods: 2 to 3 servings daily
- Fruit and vegetables: 8 to 10 servings daily
- Meat, poultry or fish: 2 or fewer 75-g (3-oz) portions daily
- Nuts, seeds and pulses: 4 to 5 servings per week
- Fats and oils: 2.5 teaspoons a day

risk of breast cancer (in some studies, excessive soya consumption is associated with cancer risk).

Since soya flour lacks gluten – the elastic component in wheat flour that allows bread or other baked goods to capture air so they're light and fluffy – you can't completely replace wheat flour with soya flour in recipes. 'Try replacing about one-quarter of the wheat flour with soya flour, and watch the cooking time,' says Barbara. 'The soya will make cakes moist and tender, but they will brown a little more quickly.' As a general rule, take 5 to 10 minutes off the baking time suggested in a regular recipe.

We've given you a lot to digest in this chapter (pardon the pun), but eating right is a key to your menopausal and postmenopausal health. Here, we've focused on eating to maintain your youthful figure, enhance your overall health and well-being, and ward off serious bodily illness; it can also help you to manage your moods.

But there's more to making menopause an easy transition than good eating. Exercise is equally essential in mid-life and beyond. In fact, it's probably even more important during the second half of life than it was in your early years.

If you exercise regularly, turn to Chapter 4, 'The Menopause Exercise Plan', to find a programme of exercises that are especially suited for menopause and beyond. They'll strengthen your bones, improve your overall health and help minimize menopausal symptoms. (They'll also make you look younger!) And if you're an exercise avoider, Chapter 4 presents a host of easy options that will let you slide into exercising without breaking sweat, joining a gym or buying costly, space-consuming equipment.

Chapter

3

THE MENOPAUSE EXERCISE PLAN

Wʜᴇɴ ɪᴛ ᴄᴏᴍᴇs ᴛᴏ ᴛʜᴇ ᴍᴇɴᴏᴘᴀᴜsᴇ ᴀɴᴅ ᴇxᴇʀᴄɪsᴇ, ɪᴛ' s ᴛɪᴍᴇ to use it or lose it, where muscles are concerned. 'Most women lose about one-third to one-half pound of muscle a year after the age of 35. By the time they're 80, some can't perform routine tasks, like getting up out of a chair or climbing stairs,' says Dr Miriam Nelson, director of the Center for Physical Fitness at Tufts University School of Nutrition Science and Policy and author of the bestselling books *Strong Women Stay Young* and *Strong Women Stay Slim*.

Part of this loss of strength is from ageing, 'but it's also from inactivity, and *that* you can do something about,' Dr Nelson says. Research shows that people who strength train seem to preserve their youthful body compositions very well.

Dr Nelson's own studies show that women in their fifties and sixties who do high-intensity strength training can develop strength scores more typical of women in their late thirties or forties. 'We have seen an increase in muscle mass in people even in their nineties,' she says. 'I'm not saying we are going to make a 90-year-old look like a 20-year-old, but we can see the body shape change and take on a more youthful appearance.'

If you already know that you should be exercising and are looking for a quick and easy plan, turn to 'The Menopause Exercise Programme' on page 71. But if you need further convincing, read on.

What Can Exercise Do for Me?

In addition to helping you look younger, exercise of any type can make you feel really good physically and psychologically after a stressful day. And the effects of exercise may go even deeper than that. Some researchers have shown that it can actually relieve depression and anxiety.

However, unless you're a police officer, builder, gym teacher or carpenter, your normal daily activities are not likely to make a big impact on your cardiovascular health, muscle strength and endurance, or flexibility, all of which are important for general health and fitness and for disease prevention.

So if you're like most people, you need a plan for exercise. Setting time aside in your day allows you to take care of yourself and anticipate a chance to relax and unwind. And it's a time to socialize if you participate in an exercise class.

Does It Really Matter What Type of Exercise I Choose?

Aerobic exercise, such as jogging or brisk walking for 30 minutes or more, increases your body's ability to process and utilize oxygen. It keeps your heart and lungs healthy, and it can help prevent diabetes, high blood pressure and certain types of cancers, says Dr Janet P. Wallace, professor of kinesiology and associate professor and director of adult fitness at Indiana University.

Weight training, on the other hand, is an anaerobic work-out. Your body doesn't have the same oxygen needs as it does when performing an aerobic exercise. Lifting weights builds lean muscle tissue, keeps you strong, gives you more energy and prevents bone loss – a major concern for women in their postmenopausal years.

Then there are flexibility exercises, such as yoga and stretching, to keep your muscles, ligaments and tendons limber and less susceptible to injury.

ENOUGH EXCUSES!

At school, we pleaded stomach cramps or 'forgot' our ugly gym kit to get out of PE class. Now, as grown women, we have more sophisticated excuses for getting out of working out. Below are the top 10 excuses for not exercising.

1. 'I'm too tired.'
2. 'I have a bad back/knee/ankle.'
3. 'I can't stick to a routine.'
4. 'It's so boring.'
5. 'My job/children/home obligations eat up my time.'
6. 'I never see results.'
7. 'I'm too embarrassed about my body to join a gym or walk in the park.'
8. 'I get out of breath easily and can't keep up.'
9. 'I don't know where to start.'
10. 'I'm too old.'

You can probably make up a great list of your own. But when you're finished, take it out to the garden and bury it. Then start working on your list of the 10 best reasons *to* exercise!

But do you really need to incorporate these different types of exercise into your daily routine? The answer is most likely *yes* if you want to accomplish most or all of these six goals.

Lose body fat. Aerobic exercise is one of the best ways to do it, along with diet adjustments, of course. Resistance training (also called weight training) can help, too, because building muscle mass through resistance training will bump up your resting metabolic rate. And that means you'll burn more calories throughout the day even when you're not exercising. But that works only to support or help maintain your weight-loss efforts. You're not going to see a big difference, either way, in the scales from weight training alone.

Get toned. Here's where resistance training does the job and where aerobic training doesn't. 'Regular resistance training will make your muscles denser so that you look better,' says Dr Priscilla Clarkson, a professor of exercise science. 'They'll become firm rather than flabby, which is often a concern in areas like the backs of your arms and your stomach.'

Get stronger. Appearance aside, strength training will make you stronger. Aerobics, on the other hand, won't do much to help you lift your daughter's three-year-old or carry heavy stuff without asking for help.

Build endurance. Aerobic work recruits the muscle fibres that specialize in endurance much more than resistance training does. So it makes perfect sense that aerobic exercise is the one that will help you enjoy those long hikes or bike rides.

Get a strong heart. This is a job for aerobics. It's your heart that has to pump all that oxygen to your muscles via your bloodstream when you're doing aerobic work. That's why your heart rate goes up. And that's why aerobic exercise is a proven strengthener of your cardiovascular system and a risk reducer for heart disease.

Spot train. It bears repeating. Neither aerobic exercise nor diets can target fat in any one body part for elimination. For that matter, neither can resistance training. If you could spot reduce, everyone who chewed gum would have a skinny face. But what resistance training can do – and aerobics can't – is target body parts for muscle toning. When you do toning exercises, you can say, 'I'm going to work on my thighs today.' Not so with aerobics.

The Health Connection

The immediate reward of any exercise programme is the deep satisfaction of looking good on the outside and feeling great on the inside. But if you step back and look at the big picture, exercise can help prevent heart disease, osteoporosis and other high-risk health problems of the postmenopausal years – as doctors have been telling us for years. Here is a brief summary of those benefits.

Lower Your Risk of Breast Cancer

Being overweight is linked to a higher risk of breast cancer, especially for women after menopause if they gained weight during adulthood. With that

HOW MUCH EXERCISE DO I NEED?

On average, two hours of aerobic activity will burn about 1000 calories. If your goal is weight loss, you need to burn 3500 calories to lose one pound (0.5 kg) of fat. So, if you spend 30 minutes jogging four times a week, you can knock off a pound (0.5 kg) of fat in 3½ weeks through exercise alone.

in mind, it seems an obvious assumption to assume that exercise will lower your risk of breast cancer. But in reality, the link between exercise and cancer risk is a fairly new area of research, and the results are hardly conclusive.

What we do know so far is that some studies seem to indicate that women who don't exercise and are overweight appear to have a higher risk of breast cancer than leaner women who exercise. A Norwegian study found that compared with women who didn't exercise at all, women who exercised at least four hours a week had a 37 per cent lower breast cancer risk. In other research, postmenopausal women who were moderately active (walking, gardening or doing housework several times a week) had a 50 per cent reduced risk of breast cancer compared with sedentary women. However, more research is being done to confirm similar findings.

Until then, make sure you include moderate exercise in your strategy to lower your risk of breast cancer. Almost all cancer research groups recommend that women try to stay at a healthy weight to help lower their risk – and exercise is a definite means to that goal.

Lift Yourself from Depression

Exercise can blast away fat, shave years off your figure, boost your energy and fight disease, but to say that it can prevent stress and depression altogether is a bit of a stretch. Nonetheless, research shows that regular aerobic activity can relieve symptoms of depression and significantly reduce stress – to the point where it's barely noticeable.

Experts theorize that's because regular exercise helps enhance your sense of mastery so you feel more mentally and physically in control. Also, when you're stressed-out, your body releases large amounts of cortisol and adrenaline, hormones that tense your muscles and speed your heart rate, blood pressure and breathing. Exercise keeps these hormone levels down and protects you from irritability, panic attacks, throbbing headaches, stomach-aches, ulcers and heart disease.

Research shows that regular aerobic exercise produces mood-enhancing chemicals called endorphins that keep us cheerful, bolster self-esteem and restore feelings of hopefulness in depressed women. So moving your body definitely helps. There's even evidence that exercise can reduce the amount of antidepressant medication you need to take, depending on the severity of your depression. In one four-month study, for example, researchers found that depressed men and women who walked or jogged three times a week for 45 minutes improved as much as a control group taking antidepressants.

Enjoy Heart Health

Researchers have found that exercise can give your body's systems the capacity to work as well as those of someone 20 years younger. So it's not surprising that physically active people – regardless of their bio-logical ages – have lower rates of heart disease and are less vulnerable to strokes.

If you haven't exercised for years, don't be put off: 'As soon as you start to exercise, your risk of cardiovascular problems drops by 25 per cent,' says Dr Gerald Fletcher, professor of medicine at the Mayo Clinic in Florida.

'Studies show that even if you start a regular exercise programme in your sixties, you lower your risk of heart disease for the rest of your life,' says Dr James M. Rippe, director of the Center for Clinical and Lifestyle Research at Tufts University School of Medicine and author of *Fit after Forty*. 'If you're 60 years old, you may have another 25 years left, so the quality of life during those years is something to think about.'

Don't let a heart attack hold you back. Exercise has been proven to be a great therapy. Studies have shown that people who became involved in an exercise programme after their first heart attacks were 20 to 40 per cent more likely to be alive seven years later than those who had survived heart attacks and then remained totally sedentary.

Exercise is so important that cardiologists often prescribe (not just recommend or suggest) exercise for patients with heart disease. In one study, researchers followed 68 patients who were on a waiting list for heart transplants and who also participated in a walking programme. After three to six months, the hearts of 30 patients had improved to the point that they no longer needed new hearts. Two years later, their hearts were still going strong.

How does aerobic exercise perform these miracles? It makes your heart pump more vigorously to carry extra blood and oxygen to hardworking muscles. Over time, the demands of exercise make your heart physically fit – stronger and more efficient. The heart becomes a bigger, stronger muscle that pumps more blood with each beat.

You get practical benefits as well. The well-exercised heart doesn't have to beat as fast when you do something demanding. Even though your body is stressed, your heart isn't. When non-exercisers clear the garden path after a snowstorm, for instance, their likelihood of a heart attack jumps to 107 times their normal risk! But someone who exercises five times a week has only 2.4 times the normal risk.

Bone Up on Exercise

What's true for muscle is also true for bones, Dr Nelson says. Use 'em or lose 'em. If women decide to sit back at menopause and allow nature to take its course, they can count on losing up to 20 per cent of bone mass in the first five to seven years, followed by a continuous slower loss. But exercise that stresses the bone, such as high-intensity strength training, can change that. It can actually preserve bone mass, and in some cases it even leads to a slight increase.

'Even that slight increase, or just maintaining bone mass, is important,' Dr Nelson says. 'The alternative is allowing your bones to become so brittle and weak over time that you can begin to have fractures.'

So no matter what your age, today is the day to start exercising. Even women who already have osteoporosis can strength train, as long as they start very slowly. While they probably won't regain enough bone mass to stop potential fractures, they can regain muscle strength, which will help them maintain balance and prevent falls. But Dr Nelson cautions, 'Women who have osteoporosis need to work with their doctors to develop a total programme, which includes exercise, nutritional support and perhaps drugs.'

Avoid Exercise Injuries

Given all the health benefits to be gained from exercising, the last thing you want to do is backslide with exercise-related injuries. And while injuries can happen any time, the first few weeks on any exercise programme tend to be particularly risky, says Dr Jean Reeve, a triathlete and associate professor of physical education. 'Mentally, you may be raring to go; but at the same time, your body is just getting used to the idea of regular work-outs,' she says. 'You need to slowly build up strength, especially around vulnerable knee and shoulder joints.'

If you're overweight, you need to be especially careful about high-impact activities, such as running or jumping. They could hurt your joints.

FORGET TOE TOUCHING! TRY THIS

Have you ever bent over to touch your toes and wanted to convince yourself later that the reason they seem so hard to reach is because your legs must be growing longer?

Well, take heart. According to many experts, you shouldn't feel bad if you can't touch your toes. The talent of toe touchers – who are actually in the minority – is due to bone structure and joint alignment, not just flexible muscles. Some people really can't touch their toes, full stop, and if they try too hard, they're likely to strain their lower-back muscles.

It's true that you should stretch your hamstrings and gluteals, the muscles on the backs of your upper thighs and buttocks. Keeping these muscles flexible helps you avoid back and knee injuries. But you don't have to touch your toes to stretch them. You can safely do a forward bend with your knees bent a bit – that takes the strain off your lower back. Ease gently into the stretch.

Or, if you find it comfortable, you can safely stretch these muscles by lying with your torso and buttocks flat on the floor and your legs straight up a wall at a 90-degree angle.

And if you're out of shape overall, Dr Reeve suggests that you may do better by initially steering clear of activities that require good balance and coordination, such as step aerobics. 'You're better off building up some muscle first with light resistance training and stair climbing,' she says.

If you're already suffering from an injury, take heart. You don't have to forget your entire work-out. 'You can probably continue to do certain exercises,' Dr Reeve says. 'But you may need to avoid using your injured area, or use it less strenuously. A physiotherapist can help you work out which moves to avoid until you're healed, and which exercises may actually help your injury heal faster.'

Here are four things to do as you begin your exercise programme.

Discuss your plans with your doctor. If you are aged 45 or older, or if you have back or joint problems, osteoarthritis, osteoporosis, high blood pressure or any other kind of chronic medical problem that makes you wonder if it's safe to exercise, Dr Reeve suggests that you clear your plans with your doctor first. If necessary, your doctor can suggest activities that you need to avoid.

Start like a tortoise, not a hare. Begin with a routine that is suited to your level of fitness. 'For people who haven't exercised in a long time, start slow and easy,' says Dr Michelle F. Mottola, an associate professor of anatomy and kinesiology. You'll beef things up as you progress. If you're lifting weights, for example, you may find that two-pound (just under one kilogram) weights are all you can handle when you start. Eventually, you'll get the weights up to the point where doing 16 repetitions is the most you can manage.

Warm up and cool down. Older bodies take time to get in the mood for exercise, get more blood flowing into muscles and limber up, Dr Nelson says. Conversely, they also need more time to slow heart rate and cool off after a work-out. A proper warm-up helps reduce your risk of injuries because it helps your muscles work at their optimal level. And, along with a cool-down, it's mandatory if you have heart disease. You can get light-headed or have chest pains from angina if you start or stop too quickly. And some drugs for high blood pressure or heart disease make your body warm up and cool down more slowly than normal. A five- to ten-minute warm-up is adequate for most people, on or off medication.

However, if you're feeling particularly stiff or sluggish, give yourself a few more minutes.

Rest. Give your muscles 48 hours between sessions to recover. Strength training two or three times a week is great for women of all ages, Dr Nelson says. 'Even older women can recover within 48 hours,' she says. If you don't recover within this period of time, you are doing too much during your sessions. You'll know that you overdid it if you are still very stiff and it's painful to move your muscles through their full range of motion.

Adjust Your Exercise Attitude

According to a study from the UK, we burn about 800 fewer calories per day than we did in 1970, mostly because of automation and labour-saving devices.

MOVING TOO MUCH

There *is* such a thing as exercising too much, says personal trainer Jana Angelakis. If you're so sore the next day that you can hardly move, you're working too hard. Becoming ill is another sign that you should cut back on your work-outs. Knowing when to stop means you're listening to your body so you won't hurt yourself, and you'll stay healthy and energized. Here are a few more red flags.

- Your performance has decreased.
- Your form and technique have deteriorated.
- You need more recovery time than usual.
- You experience a loss of appetite.
- You feel fatigued or nauseated during work-outs.
- You get headaches during work-outs.

If you experience such symptoms as undue breathlessness, light-headedness, chest pains and an irregular heartbeat, you could just be overdoing it with exercise, but you should consult a doctor to be sure.

'Physical activity has been pushed out of our lives,' says Dr Nelson. 'This means we have to choose ways to work activity back into our lives. We have to consciously get up more, walk more, take the stairs more. Whenever possible, we need to seek out activity.'

Find the Time

Most moderate-intensity activities – walking briskly, raking leaves, mowing the lawn with a push mower, hoovering – will burn 150 calories in about 30 minutes. So in addition to just counting calories, add up your minutes of activity each day. To lose weight and keep it off, you actually need about 60 minutes of activity a day, according to the latest research.

It doesn't make any difference if you do it all at once or break it up into smaller chunks of time. Everything counts.

Here are a few ways to motivate yourself to get those 60 minutes in each day.

Step up the intensity. Michelle Edwards, a health expert and personal trainer, advises her clients to start by simply increasing the intensity of any physical activity that they're already doing. That can mean taking the stairs a little faster, choosing parking spaces at the far end of the car park, or making wider arm circles when wiping off the kitchen counter. The idea is to put a little more effort into every activity in order to burn more calories.

Keep a diary. For the next few days, clock yourself every time you walk, clean, garden, climb a flight of stairs or perform any other activity that involves moving the muscles in your arms and legs. At the end of the day, add up your active time. This helps create a vivid picture of how the minutes add up, explains Michelle. Once you do this, you'll probably find yourself thinking of all kinds of ways to add a few more minutes here and there throughout the day.

One of the keys to becoming more active is learning to identify opportunities in your day and taking advantage of them. 'Five minutes here; 10 minutes there. It all adds up,' she says.

It also helps to record how much time you spend sitting each day,

WHY DO I HATE TO EXERCISE?

No woman 'hates' to exercise. What she hates are her preconceived notions about exercise – that it's painful and inconvenient, that she doesn't do it correctly, that it's a chore rather than an activity that can be both fun and beneficial to her physical and emotional well-being, that she looks ridiculous in exercise clothes.

When women associate exercise with physical pain, it's often because they lifted more weight than they should have or did too many repetitions during their first visits to the gym. When they couldn't move the next day, they blamed the exercise itself, rather than an over-ambitious work-out.

Other women think they dislike exercise because they feel foolish doing it. They think that it requires physical skill or feel pressured to exercise flawlessly, much in the way they feel pressured to be perfect mothers or perfect workers. But doing an arm curl or leg extension doesn't require any unique skills whatsoever.

Women may also hate working out because they believe it should be unpleasant or boring – that if it feels good, it can't possibly have any serious benefits. But, as many women who have 'hated' exercise have learned, exercise comes in many different forms. You just have to find the form that works for you, whether it's Pilates or power yoga, kickboxing or cycling in the park.

If you 'hate' to exercise, challenge your assumptions about it. Then try to reframe your idea of exercise in a positive light. Think of it as a gift from you to yourself, as a time-out from the hustle and bustle of your daily life.

Remember, too, that it takes some time to make exercise a habit – at least six weeks. If you can stick to an exercise programme for that long, you may find that far from 'hating' exercise, you actually look forward to your work-outs.

and to do the reverse. Work out ways to gradually replace the sitting with activity.

Get a pedometer. If you want to get a clearer picture of the amount of physical activity you are doing in a day, record how many steps you take on an average day and then find ways to add more. Studies show that people who are active for 30 minutes each day accumulate about 10,000 steps, while the average person who works in an office typically takes about 2,000 to 4,000 steps a day. 'A pedometer can be a motivational tool, a way to self-monitor,' says Michelle. 'And we know from experience that people who self-monitor are more likely to reach their activity goals than people who do not.'

Be prepared. Keep walking shoes in your car or at your desk so that you can walk whenever you have a few minutes.

Schedule it. We tend to keep our appointments, so make an appointment to exercise. You can start by scheduling exercise in the morning instead of later in the day, suggests Dr Denise Bruner, president of the American Society of Bariatric Physicians (a group of doctors who specialize in weight-loss treatments). 'Women seem to be more successful in general if they put activity on the front end of the day, versus the end of the day, when either work-related issues or home issues can end up taking precedence over exercise time,' she says.

The Menopause Exercise Programme

As we've already said, all forms of exercise give you more energy. And for optimal energy, you need a programme that combines cardiovascular activity, strength and toning exercises, and stretching. So wouldn't it be great to have one work-out that does all those things and lasts no longer than an episode of your favourite sitcom? Well, here it is!

Our Menopause Exercise Programme for total body toning is a muscle-toning, strength-training programme specially designed to raise your heart rate and increase your flexibility. You get all your fitness benefits rolled into one fat-blasting 25-minute routine.

The concept behind this plan is circuit training, and it works like this. You have a series of strength-training exercises, which you perform back-to-back with little rest in between. Like traditional strength training, circuit training builds muscle, which helps you to burn more calories when you're not exercising.

In addition, circuit training gives you a cardio work-out. Because you move quickly from one exercise to the next, your heart rate stays up, and you burn more calories while you're lifting weights.

To add flexibility benefits – an essential fitness component, especially as you get older – we've mixed in a few yoga poses. These easy moves

BURNING CALORIES

If you are a 67-kg (10½ st) woman, how long does it take to burn 150 calories? That depends on what you do. (If you weigh more, it may take less intensity to burn the same number of calories.)

Ironing	59 minutes
Cooking	48 minutes
Washing and waxing a car	45 to 60 minutes
Playing volleyball	45 minutes
Strolling through the shopping centre	44 minutes
Grocery shopping	36 minutes
Doing yoga	36 minutes
Hoovering	34 minutes
Gardening	30 to 45 minutes
Cycling leisurely	30 minutes
Brisk walking	30 minutes
Dancing fast	30 minutes
Pushing a pushchair	30 minutes
Raking leaves	30 minutes
Mowing the lawn with a push mower	29 minutes
Rollerblading leisurely	26 minutes
Stacking firewood	25 minutes
Bowling	23 minutes
House-cleaning	21 minutes
Scrubbing floors	20 minutes
Swimming	19 minutes
Climbing stairs	15 minutes
Shovelling snow	15 minutes

stretch your muscles while also helping to further increase your strength. (Research shows that stretching while you lift weights can boost strength gains by 20 per cent.)

'With circuit training, you can get a good cardiovascular work-out and great muscle definition in a short time,' says Vern Gambetta a coach who trains Olympic and professional athletes using circuit training.

The Menopause Exercise Programme Basics

The exercises in our circuits are bunched into groups of three, followed by a stretch. Perform each exercise for 60 seconds, doing as many repetitions as possible. (It helps to have a clock with a second hand or a timer nearby.)

LIFTING WEIGHTS VERSUS JOGGING

Research has shown that when volunteers performed just 20 minutes of circuit training three days a week, they improved their fitness levels by up to 11 per cent. That's about the same cardiovascular boost a similar group got when they jogged for 30 minutes, three days a week.

More recently, researchers found that when previously sedentary adults did 40 minutes of either circuit training or endurance exercise, such as cycling or cross-country skiing, three days a week, both groups had similar aerobic benefits, with the circuit trainers reaping the added benefit of increased muscle strength.

Another advantage of circuit training is that it's fun. That's because you're constantly moving to a new exercise, which keeps it interesting.

Circuit 1

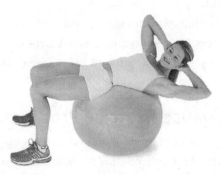

1. Twisting crunch on a ball: sit on an exercise ball with your feet on the floor, shoulder-width apart. Place your fingertips lightly behind your head. Lean back (the ball will roll forwards slightly) so your rear and the small of your back are pressing against the ball. Use your abdominal muscles to lift your shoulders up and forwards, twisting your right shoulder towards your left side as you lift. Pause, then lower. Repeat, alternating sides, for a total of 60 seconds. Rest for 15 seconds before moving on to the next exercise.

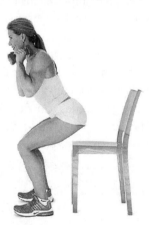

2. Dumbbell squat: stand with your back to a chair, your feet about shoulder-width apart. Hold the dumbbells at your shoulders, palms facing in. Keeping your back straight, bend at the knees and hips as though you were sitting down. Don't let your knees move forwards beyond your toes. Stop just short of touching the chair, then stand up. Repeat for 60 seconds. Rest for 15 seconds before moving on to the next exercise.

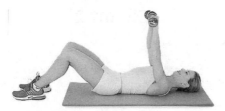

3. Chest press: lying on the floor (or a bench), hold the dumbbells end to end just above chest height; your elbows should be pointing out. Press the dumbbells straight up, extending your arms. Hold, then lower. Repeat for 60 seconds. Rest 15 seconds before moving on to the next exercise.

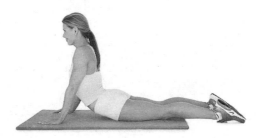

4. Cobra stretch: lie face down with your feet together, your toes pointed, and your hands on the floor, palms down just in front of your shoulders. Press your hands into the floor and gently extend your arms, lifting your upper body as far as is comfortably possible. If you feel any strain in your back, alter the pose so that you keep your elbows bent and your palms on the floor. Hold for 15 seconds.

Circuit 2

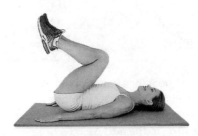

1. Reverse curl: lie on your back with your arms at your sides, palms down. Bend your hips and knees so that your legs are over your mid-section and relaxed. Slowly contract your abdominal muscles, lifting your hips 5–10 cm (2–4 in) off the floor. Hold, then slowly lower. Repeat for 60 seconds. Rest for 15 seconds before moving on to the next exercise.

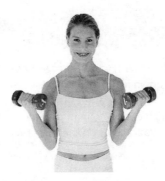

2. Biceps curl: stand with your feet shoulder-width apart, holding dumbbells at your sides. Bending your elbows and turning your wrists upward, lift the dumbbells towards your shoulders. Don't move your upper arms. Stop when the dumbbells are at chest height, palms facing your body. Pause, then lower. Repeat for 60 seconds. Rest for 15 seconds before moving on to the next exercise.

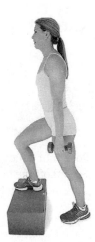

3. Step up: stand facing an aerobic step or regular stairs, holding dumbbells at your sides. Place your right foot on the step, and lift yourself up. Just tap your left foot on the top of the step, slowly lower your left foot to the floor, then step off with your right foot. Repeat, alternating feet, for a total of 60 seconds. Rest for 15 seconds before moving on to the next exercise.

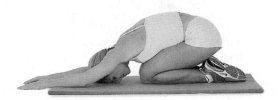

4. Praise pose stretch: kneel with your toes pointed behind you. Sit back onto your heels, and lower your chest to your thighs. Stretch your arms overhead, and rest your palms and forehead on the floor (or as close as is comfortable). Hold for 15 seconds.

Circuit 3

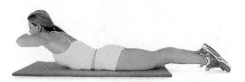

1. Chest lift: lie face down on the floor, your hands under your chin. Lift your head, chest and arms about 12–15 cm (5–6 in) off the floor. Hold, then lower. Repeat for 60 seconds. Rest for 15 seconds before moving on to the next exercise.

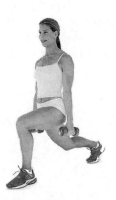

2. Lunge: stand with your feet together, holding dumbbells down at your sides, your palms facing in. Take one big step forwards with your left leg. Plant your left foot, then slowly lower your right knee towards the floor. Your left knee should be at a 90-degree angle, your back straight. Press into your left foot, and push yourself back to the starting position. Repeat, alternating legs, for a total of 60 seconds. Rest for 15 seconds before moving on to the next exercise.

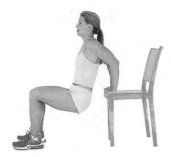

3. Dip: sit on the edge of a sturdy chair, hands grasping the seat on either side of your bottom. Walk your feet out slightly, and inch your bottom off the chair. Keeping your shoulders down and your back straight, bend your elbows back, and lower your bottom towards the floor as far as is comfortably possible. Slowly push back up. Repeat for 60 seconds. Rest for 15 seconds before moving on to the next exercise.

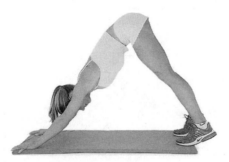

4. Downward dog stretch: position yourself on the floor on your hands and knees, with your feet flexed. Press your hands and feet into the floor, raising your hips towards the ceiling. Your body should look like an upside-down V. Keep lifting your tailbone towards the ceiling as you lower your heels to the floor as far as is comfortably possible. Hold for 15 seconds.

Circuit 4

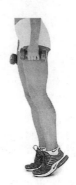

1. Calf raise: stand with your feet about hip-width apart, holding dumbbells at your sides. Slowly rise onto your toes while keeping your torso and legs straight. Hold, then lower. Repeat for 60 seconds. Rest for 15 seconds before moving on to the next exercise.

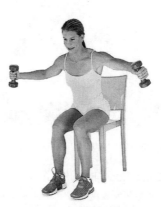

2. Back fly: sit in a chair, your feet flat on the floor and about hip-width apart. Hold a dumbbell in each hand so the weights are about chest level and about 30 cm (12 in) from your body. Your palms should be facing each other and your elbows slightly bent as if you were holding a beach ball. Bend forwards from the hips about 7–12 cm (3–5 in). Keeping your back straight, squeeze your shoulder blades together, and pull your elbows back as far as is comfortably possible. Pause, then return to the starting position. Repeat for 60 seconds. Rest for 15 seconds before moving on to the next exercise.

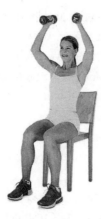

3. Overhead press: sit in a chair, your feet flat on the floor. Hold dumbbells up at shoulder height, your palms facing your ears. Press the dumbbells straight overhead without locking your elbows. Hold, then lower. Repeat for 60 seconds. Rest for 15 seconds before moving on to the next exercise.

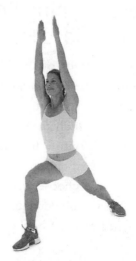

4. Warrior stretch: stand tall, your feet about hip-width apart. Take a giant step forwards with your right foot, bending that knee. (Be sure your knee does not jut out over your toes.) Turn your left foot to the side so your left arch faces the heel of your right foot. Raise your arms over your head, your palms facing each other, your chin slightly lifted. Hold for 15 seconds, then switch sides.

You can use a lighter weight and perform more repetitions – or a heavier weight and perform fewer, slower repetitions – so long as you maintain good form and challenge yourself. The effort should feel tough during the final 10 to 15 seconds. To avoid injury, allow at least three seconds to lift and three seconds to lower the weight for each repetition.

Rest no more than 15 seconds between exercises. Before you start, always warm up with 5 minutes of moderate exercise, such as walking or stationary cycling. When you've finished, cool down with five minutes of easy activity.

Use this work-out three days a week, and you'll see results in as little as four weeks. You'll get even greater results if you make it part of a cross-training, variety-packed programme. For instance, you might try circuit training Monday, Wednesday and Friday, cycling on Tuesdays, walking on Thursdays and hiking in the country at weekends. For more cross-training ideas, see opposite.

Create a Cross-training Programme – and Have Fun

In order to speed up the results of the Menopause Exercise Programme, try to work in other fitness activities on the days that you don't circuit train. It really doesn't matter what you do, as long as you choose an activity that you enjoy. You might try singles tennis, cross-country skiing, swimming, a brisk walk with a friend, or rollerblading or ice-skating. We've compiled a menu of options to get you started.

Regardless of the activity you choose, make sure you start at a comfortable speed and gradually increase your intensity within five minutes. You should break into a light sweat and be slightly breathless but still able to hold a conversation.

Walking. Everyone knows that walking is as simple as putting one foot in front of the other. But if you want to lose weight, you'll have to walk like a woman on a mission – and pump your arms. In other words, power walk.

If you power walk regularly, your body will burn more calories and fat

CIRCUIT TRICKS

To make your circuit work-outs feel more like play than work, try these circuit tricks during your next session.

Perform to a soundtrack. Because it's rhythmic and consistent, circuit training works well to music. Pick a CD with a steady beat that will keep you humming along. Anything R&B works well.

Form a circuit circle. First there were sewing circles, then book groups. Invite a friend or two to work out with you. Each person starts at a different point in the circuit; every 60 seconds, shout 'Change!' and move to the next exercise.

Do the shuffle. Keep the work-out fresh and interesting by changing the order whenever it feels too familiar. Since the exercises are bundled in groups of three followed by a stretch, just rearrange the groups, one week starting with group two, the next week group three, and so on.

throughout the day because of the boost to your metabolism. You'll firm up the muscles in your buttocks, thighs, calves, back, upper arms, shoulders and abdomen. You'll condition your cardiovascular system; reduce stress, heart disease and stroke risk; help prevent osteoporosis; and elevate your mood. On average, walking burns 100 calories per 1.6 km (1 mile), so you can burn 350 to 450 calories an hour, depending on how fast you walk and whether you hike on flat or hilly terrain.

Step aerobics. Choreographed to the beat of heart-pumping music, step aerobics are high-intensity, low-impact exercises that combine dance moves on and around an adjustable platform. The 'step' exploded onto the fitness scene in the late 1980s and hasn't lost its popularity yet.

Aerobics can help tone and shape the muscles in your buttocks, hips, thighs, calves and abs. Plus, the arm movements will sculpt your biceps, triceps and shoulders. Depending on the intensity of your work-out, you can burn 600 calories in an hour using a 15-cm (6-in) step.

Jogging. Like walking, jogging is one of the most accessible – and enjoyable – aerobic activities. But that's where the similarities end. While jogging burns about the same number of calories per mile, you're moving a lot faster than with walking, so you burn calories faster, too (about 500

EAT FOR SUCCESS

What you eat can speed up – or slow down – your success. For the best results from the Menopause Exercise Programme for total-body toning, try this advice.

Start with a snack. Too many women exercise on empty, hoping they'll burn more calories and lose more weight. The reality is that you don't perform as well and can't lift as much when you're not well-fuelled, so the work-out is less effective.

If it's been more than two to three hours since your last meal, eat a small snack, such as a banana, about 30 minutes before lifting. Just make sure that you compensate for these additional calories (110 for a medium banana) by cutting back a little at a later meal.

Pump up your protein. Protein helps to repair your working muscles after a bout of lifting weights so that they get stronger. To make sure you're getting enough, plan on eating about ½ gram of protein per 0.5 kg (1 lb) of body weight. So a 64 kg (10 st) woman would aim for 70 grams of protein a day.

Make sure with a multi. People who exercise regularly have a higher demand for many vitamins and minerals than do sedentary people. The best way to get them is to eat more fruit and vegetables. Experts recommend at least five a day. It's also a good idea to take a standard multivitamin for insurance.

to 600 calories per hour). And afterwards, your metabolic rate stays supercharged for hours.

In addition to strengthening and toning your abs and the muscles in your buttocks, hips, thighs and calves, jogging is one of the quickest ways to achieve cardiovascular fitness.

Spinning. You'll be glad to know that twirling around in circles like a top is not the work-out we're talking about here. Spinning is an aerobic, high-intensity indoor cycling class that conditions your cardiovascular system and tones the muscles in your thighs, calves, buttocks and hips. With upbeat music playing in the background, an instructor takes you through a routine that challenges you with intervals of fast and slow riding at various speeds and resistances. Throughout the work-out, she helps you to imagine yourself riding through hill climbs, fast descents and all kinds of thrilling cycling scenarios. And you'll burn 260 to 660 calories an hour, depending on your weight and how intensely you pedal.

Classes are held at most gyms. You can buy your own exercise bike

WHATEVER HAPPENED TO CALLISTHENICS?

It's easy to have mixed feelings about callisthenics. On the one hand, the word comes from two Greek roots meaning 'beauty' and 'strength'—qualities that are certainly worth saving from extinction! On the other, it will forever be associated with that sadistic PE teacher you had at school. No wonder it's an endangered exercise species.

Callisthenics usually refers to an exercise routine that you do without weights or any other equipment. Well-known callisthenics movements include push-ups, sit-ups, jumping jacks, running on the spot and leg lifts.

You can see from that partial list that callisthenics haven't entirely disappeared. The 'legwork' that is tacked on to many aerobics classes is a lot like callisthenics. In any weight-training routine, work-outs for your midsection will consist mostly of crunches and similar exercises. And push-ups are still considered a pretty good upper-body strengthener.

Certain traditional callisthenics movements, however, have turned out to do more harm than good. Deep knee bends are a prime example. That's one reason why callisthenics have been declining in popularity. Another is those negative associations. Yet another is that — let's face it — callisthenics are boring. And if you really want to be cynical, you can blame their demise on the fact that it's pretty hard to sell merchandise around such an equipment-free, no-frills mode of exercise.

But the main reason that you don't hear too much about callisthenics these days is that we've found better ways to get fit. In the last few decades, new knowledge about aerobic exercise has pushed jumping jacks into dinosaur land. More importantly (since strength and toning is the main goal of callisthenics), resistance training has been shown to get results more quickly, more thoroughly and more easily than any callisthenics routine. Weights let you adjust the resistance so you can make steady progress. Weights also let you concentrate on individual muscles in a way that callisthenics can't.

And yes, weight training is a lot more fun.

designed for spinning and work out in the comfort of your own home. But without the direction of a fitness trainer, you may not burn as many calories – or have as much fun. It's the environment you're in that makes spinning such great exercise. The instructor pushes you, the music pushes you, and the people in the class push you.

Kickboxing. The word may conjure up images of spindly martial arts champions waiting to knock out their opponents, but at your local health club or leisure centre, kickboxing is a non-contact cardiovascular work-out that combines aerobic exercise with shadowboxing to whip you into ringside shape. A total-body cardiovascular work-out, kickboxing sculpts and tones your arms, back, hips, thighs, calves and abs and can improve your sense of coordination and balance.

Essentially, it involves a series of kicking, punching and blocking movements against an imaginary opponent that are choreographed to high-energy music. Classes often go by the names Kwando, Cardio Kickboxing, Cardio Kicks, Boxercise, Tae-Bo or just kickboxing. Depending on the club, you may wear boxing gloves or hand mitts, use actual punch bags or combine the movements with step aerobics. You can also buy or rent kickboxing videotapes and do the routines at home. Either way, you can burn 680 or more calories in a one-hour session.

Table tennis. If you have a table tennis table packed away in your cellar or garage somewhere, take it out, dust it off and call a friend. Hitting a small lightweight ball back and forth across a table actually counts as a real work-out because it strengthens your quadriceps, hamstrings, inner and outer thighs and hips.

Plus, you can burn 270 calories per hour of steady playing. The type of work-out you get is directly related to the level of skill with which you and your partner play. If you really want to start incinerating some calories and improving your game, find a friend who would like to practise a minimum of three times a week for about an hour each time. Some tables fold up on one side so that you can play by yourself against the upended tabletop – a handy option if you can't find someone else to play as regularly as you'd like.

Feeling motivated? Great! Head for the gym, go for a walk or climb on the exercise bike right now. Once you're back, cooled down and ready to relax, turn to Chapter 5 to find out all about the best supplements to help you stay healthy through menopause and beyond.

Chapter

4

SUPER MENOPAUSE SUPPLEMENTS

Eₓₚₑᵣₜₛ ᴀssuʀᴇ us ᴛʜᴀᴛ ᴍᴇɴopᴀusᴇ ɪs ᴀ ᴛɪᴍᴇ ᴏꜰ ʟɪꜰᴇ, ɴᴏᴛ ᴀ disease that can be 'cured'. If only it were that easy. Yes, we certainly agree: menopause is not a disease. But the hormonal ebb and flow that characterizes the years before and during menopause creates a flood of symptoms that range from merely irritating to totally debilitating. And after menopause, women are at higher risk for three major diseases: heart disease, cancer (especially endometrial and breast cancers) and osteoporosis.

If you're like us, you'll want to do everything possible to strengthen your body against this onslaught – and that's where supplements can help. By making sure you're getting the right combination and amounts of vitamins, minerals and other supplements, you can give your body a powerful weapon to ward off menopause's worst effects. And luckily doctors, herbalists and other experts now know quite a lot about what to take specifically for menopause, as you'll see in this chapter.

What you choose to take depends on your situation, so we present the information in this chapter to help you customize a supplement programme that meets your individual needs. We recommend that all women take the basic vitamins and minerals in the section called 'Restoring Your Balance' on the opposite page. Menopause brings with it a lot of long-term mental, physical and emotional stress. A well--nourished, well-rested, carefully supplemented body can help you minimize stress in all three areas.

If you find yourself experiencing uncomfortable or embarrassing menopausal symptoms turn to 'Menopausal Changes' on page 93, look up your symptom, and choose one or more of the supplements we suggest to combat it. And if you have a family history of or have personally experienced heart disease, cancer or osteoporosis, you should read all your options in 'Healing the Heart' on page 109, 'Combating Cancer' on page 117 and 'Outwitting Osteoporosis' on page 125.

To make it easier for you to remember what you'd like to take, we've included Super Supplement Checklists throughout the chapter. You can photocopy the ones that interest you (say, the ones on general supplements, menopausal symptoms and osteoporosis), then tick off the supplements you feel would be most helpful to you as you read about them in the chapter. We recommend that when you're finished making your list, but before you begin your shopping excursion, you discuss with your doctor the supplements you'd like to take. Then take your checklists to the healthfood shop, chemist or supermarket, and see at a glance what you need to buy. You may also find a wider variety by shopping on the internet. For more on supplements, see Chapter 9.

Restoring Your Balance

Menopause is kind of like puberty in reverse. In puberty, your body started producing larger quantities of the hormones oestrogen and progesterone, among others, and you started to menstruate. In menopause, your body produces less of these hormones, so you stop menstruating.

By now, your body has become used to higher hormone levels. Thus, for some women, menopause is like putting your body through withdrawal. Here are some supplements that can provide you with a good foundation for stemming the tides of time and helping you look and feel younger.

Multivitamin/mineral supplement. This is an easy way to make sure that you're getting enough of all the nutrients your body needs: folic acid, vitamins B_6 and B_{12}, chromium, selenium and magnesium. As we age, we absorb less of the nutrients than we once did. We also tend to eat less, so a multivitamin is a great way to supplement your diet with the essentials. Look for a 'mega' supplement that has 600 to 1,000 per cent of the RDA (recommended daily allowance) for all your B vitamins, 100 to 200 milligrams of vitamin C, and a good spread of trace minerals, says Dr Connie Catellani, an expert in integrative medicine.

Note that only women who are still having periods or who are anaemic should take iron supplements. (Acids increase iron absorption, so take your iron with some orange juice.) If you aren't anaemic and are past childbearing age, look for an iron-free multivitamin/mineral formulation. (Most supplements targeted at men are iron-free, and more general iron-free supplements are becoming available.)

Vitamin C with bioflavonoids. As an antioxidant, vitamin C plays an important role in preventing disease. Antioxidants are protective substances that help destroy unstable molecules that can damage cells and make them more susceptible to cancer. Vitamin C also helps to lower blood pressure, which could also protect your arteries and heart. Bioflavonoids are compounds found in citrus fruit that have be shown to protect capillaries and other small blood vessels.

Vitamin E. Vitamin E is very important for heart health. If your multivitamin supplement contains 200 international units (IU) or so, take an additional 200 to 400 IU as a separate supplement. Like vitamin C,

SUPER SUPPLEMENT CHECKLIST No. 1

Here's a checklist for general supplementation. Choose these supplements to help yourself stay in peak nutritional health throughout the menopausal years, from perimenopause straight through to postmenopause.

- ☐ 'Mega' multivitamin/mineral supplement
- ☐ Vitamin C with bioflavonoids
- ☐ Vitamin E
- ☐ Calcium
- ☐ Vitamin D

VITAMIN D:
THE 'OTHER' BONE-FRIENDLY HORMONE

Way back in 1922, at the University of Wisconsin, professor Elmer McCollum discovered vitamin D in cod liver oil, earning himself the title 'Father of Vitamin D'. Over 80 years later, vitamin D is still a hot research topic at the university, where three generations of scientists have studied the nutrient.

Leading the latest wave of researchers is Dr Hector DeLuca, chair of the biochemistry department, who has studied vitamin D since 1951. Five decades later, he remains intrigued by this vitamin and its benefits in the body.

Technically, vitamin D is a hormone, not a vitamin, says Dr DeLuca. And while oestrogen gets all the attention for protecting your bones, your body relies on vitamin D to fully absorb calcium, keep bones strong and prevent osteoporosis. Vitamin D targets the intestines, kidneys and bones, all of which respond by making calcium available for bone growth.

'In a sense, vitamin D acts like a chauffeur, driving calcium to where it is needed in the body,' says Dr DeLuca. 'I believe all life originated in the sea, where calcium was abundant. Today we live on land, where calcium is not so abundant. I think vitamin D has evolved to help us with this calcium shortage.'

Even if you drink milk, eat yoghurt or other calcium-fortified foods, and take calcium supplements, you need to make sure you're getting enough vitamin D

vitamin E is an antioxidant and thus is important in the fight against ageing and cancer.

Calcium and vitamin D. The calcium in your bones is like savings in a bank. You deposit calcium through the foods you eat, and when your body needs calcium – which it uses for many important functions, such as regulating muscle contraction, heartbeat and blood clotting – it's 'withdrawn' from the bones. If withdrawals exceed deposits, bones eventually weaken and become fragile. Most of us begin to lose bone around the age of 35, but additional calcium may help slow that loss. The best way to meet your calcium needs is through various foods and drinks. However, older people, as well as people who consume few dairy products, may need to supplement.

Just as important to bone health is vitamin D, which your body needs

– 400 International Units a day – especially in winter, says Dr DeLuca. Your body uses sunlight to produce vitamin D. So spending as little as 10 minutes a day in the summer sun is enough to soak up a whole day's worth of D. Using sunscreen will interfere with the production of vitamin D, however, and sunblock will completely prevent it. Yet you don't want to forgo protection during peak hours. The best solution: drink in those rays after 3 pm, when the sun isn't so damaging, and wear sunblock the rest of the time.

If you live in cold countries, squeezing out even 200 IU of vitamin D from the sun can be difficult, however. 'If it's cold and snowy for weeks, and you don't get out, your vitamin D may be totally depleted by April,' says Dr DeLuca. Sunlight pouring through a window won't do because glass filters out the rays you need most for vitamin D. If you're not sure you're getting enough vitamin D, Dr DeLuca recommends taking a supplement once a day that provides 400 IU of vitamin D, along with the recommended intake of 1,000 to 1,200 milligrams of calcium.

Avoid taking more than the recommended amount of vitamin D. Taking large amounts – 2,000 IU or more of vitamin D a day over several months – can cause high blood levels of calcium, kidney damage, and calcium deposits in the heart and lungs, which can be fatal. And if you take combination calcium/vitamin D supplements, make sure you keep your daily calcium intake under 2,500 milligrams.

in order to use calcium. Unfortunately, many women aged 50 or older don't get enough to keep their bones strong. You should be getting 1,200 milligrams a day of calcium, including supplements if necessary, and 400 to 800 IU a day of vitamin D if you are aged 50 or over.

Menopausal Changes

The changes that arise around the time of menopause may be predictable, but that certainly doesn't make them comfortable. Hot flushes and night sweats are just the beginning. Women may also experience vaginal dryness, loss of sex drive, mood swings, depression and a host of related problems.

There are a number of herbs and supplements that may help. Some address the whole range of discomforts, while others take aim at specific problems, such as vaginal dryness or low sex drive. Here is an overview of what these supplements can do for you.

Hot Flushes and Night Sweats

While we don't really know what causes hot flushes, we do know that as many as 65 to 80 per cent of women will experience them at some point during their transition to menopause. Whatever the cause, hot flushes are uncomfortable and unpredictable, sometimes disturbing a restful night's sleep. You wake drenched in sweat, sometimes several times a night – hence the name 'night sweats'. Because night sweats disturb sleep, you're often tired during the day. Here are some suggestions to help you chill out.

Vitamin E. About 400 IU of vitamin E a day helps decrease hot flushes by balancing the levels of oestrogen in your body. Not only that, but research shows that postmenopausal women who get at least this much vitamin E have a lower risk of death from heart disease. Getting enough vitamin E from a low-fat diet is a bit difficult. So take a vitamin E supplement with a little bit of fat to ensure absorption. It may not work right away, however. You may have to take vitamin E for at least six weeks before noticing any effects.

Vitamin C and bioflavonoids. Research has found that by strengthening and stabilizing capillaries and other small blood vessels, these supplements in combination can prevent hot flushes from occurring. You can find supplements that combine vitamin C and bioflavonoids at most healthfood shops. Look for a supplement that contains 500 to 1,000 milligrams of vitamin C, and 200 to 500 milligrams of bioflavonoids, per capsule.

Pantothenic acid. This B vitamin boosts the functions of your adrenal glands, which take over most of the oestrogen production when your reproductive system stops. If night sweats are causing insomnia, try taking 500 milligrams a day. Continue to take it until you get relief.

Black cohosh. This herb (*Actaea racemosa*) has oestrogen-like effects, which enable it to quell hot flushes. Several clinical trials found that black cohosh reduced hot flushes by up to 80 per cent. To put your fire out, take

SUPER SUPPLEMENT CHECKLIST No. 2

If you're experiencing unpleasant menopause symptoms, here's an array of supplements to help you, organized by symptom. (Remember, we're not advising you to take them all at once! Read the descriptions of each and their effects, then pick the ones you think would work best for your situation.)

Hot Flushes and Night Sweats
- [ ] Vitamin E
- [ ] Vitamin C with bioflavonoids
- [ ] Pantothenic acid
- [ ] Black cohosh
- [ ] Flaxseed (Linseed)
- [ ] Sage
- [ ] Angelica sinensis, damiana and agnus castus
- [ ] Motherwort and agnus castus

Irregular Periods and Flooding
- [ ] Iron
- [ ] Yellow dock root
- [ ] Vitamin C with bioflavonoids
- [ ] Agnus castus
- [ ] Black cohosh
- [ ] Cinnamon
- [ ] Angelica sinensis
- [ ] Lady's mantle

Vaginal Dryness
- [ ] Liquorice
- [ ] Panax ginseng
- [ ] Black cohosh and Angelica sinensis

Mood Swings
- [ ] Calcium
- [ ] Magnesium and vitamin B_6
- [ ] Pantothenic acid
- [ ] Black cohosh
- [ ] Chamomile
- [ ] Skullcap
- [ ] Agnus castus

4 milligrams of black cohosh, either in one dose or in two 2-milligram tablets twice a day, but don't use it for more than six months.

Flaxseed (Linseed). Flaxseed's essential fatty acids act like weak oestrogens in your body, helping to relieve menopausal symptoms and lubricate vaginal tissues, writes Dr Lana Lew, an Australian women's health specialist, in her book *The Natural Oestrogen Diet*. Flaxseed also contains omega-3 fatty acids, which help protect your heart. You need to take 1 to

2 tablespoons of flaxseed a day to get the greatest benefit. Because your body can't absorb the healing properties of the whole seeds, buy ground flaxseeds at healthfood shops, or grind them in a coffee grinder. To get what you need each day, add a tablespoon to your cereal in the morning and another to yoghurt, baked goods or salads.

Sage. Garden sage is famed for the way it reduces or even eliminates night sweats. It acts fast – within a few hours – and a single cup of infusion can stave off the sweats for up to two days, says Susun S. Weed, a herbalist and author of the *Wise Woman* series of herbal health books. What's more, you probably have a jar of sage sitting on your spice rack. Just make sure it's still nice and aromatic before you use it medicinally.

To make a sage infusion, put 4 heaped tablespoons of dried sage in a mug or jam jar of hot water. Cover tightly and steep for four hours or more. Strain and drink hot or cold. Or, for a no-fuss infusion, look for sage tea bags at your healthfood shop.

Herbal combinations. 'My own standard recommendation for hot flushes and other symptoms of menopause is a trio of traditional herbs,' says Dr Andrew Weil, director of the programme in integrative medicine at the University of Arizona College of Medicine and author of *Spontaneous Healing*. Dr Weil recommends taking 1 dropperful each of tinctures of Angelica sinensis (also known as Chinese angelica or dong gui), agnus castus (also called vitex) and damiana once a day at midday. Continue taking the herbs until your hot flushes cease, then taper off gradually.

Angelica sinensis is a herb that has been used for centuries in China.

DON'T USE HRT AND BLACK COHOSH TOGETHER

Using prescription hormone replacement therapy (HRT) and black cohosh together is not recommended. 'Both of them work on your endocrine system, so it's best to err on the side of caution. Choose one or the other, but not both,' recommends herbalist Douglas Schar. 'Think of it as doubling up, using paracetamol and aspirin together for a headache, or Tums and Rennies for indigestion.'

In fact, it is Chinese medicine's leading remedy for gynaecological ailments. Don't use Angelica sinensis while menstruating, spotting or bleeding heavily because it can increase blood loss.

Damiana is a nervous system tonic said to ease depression and anxiety. Agnus castus may counteract the effectiveness of birth control pills, so if you're on them, don't take this herb.

Motherwort and agnus castus. For some women, menopause follows surgical removal of the ovaries, or chemotherapy or radiation treatments that can destroy the ovaries. If you're one of these women, your hot flushes may be especially frequent and intense. Volcanic hot flushes are to a normal hot flush as a tidal wave is to a normal wave. Twenty-five to 30 drops of motherwort tincture can stem the tide. And for the long term, experts recommend 30 to 90 drops of agnus castus tincture three times a day for at least 13 months.

Irregular Periods and Flooding

You might call the decade before menopause 'period pause'. Your period used to arrive like clockwork, every 28 days. Now it's early one month and late the next. Sometimes it doesn't show up for months. And when it does, it may last two weeks or more. Your periods may be very heavy or very light. What's going on here?

If you're in your forties but not yet menopausal, your hormones may be on the blink. Levels of oestrogen and progesterone, which used to fluctuate on cue, may surge one month or be released at odd times the next. It's a complex change in the symphony of hormones that is being played inside a woman's body. But it's a normal passage that every woman goes through. Even so, that doesn't mean you have to put up with problem periods. Let these supplements and herbs help you to navigate the transition from super tampons to none.

Iron. If you are experiencing heavy blood loss, iron may be the most important mineral you can take to help control it. Heavy menstrual flow can deplete your body's iron stores, and some researchers also believe that chronic iron deficiency may cause heavy bleeding. Do not take more than the RNI (14.8 milligrams) on your own, though. You must be tested for iron deficiency before supplementing with higher doses.

PERIMENOPAUSAL RELIEF TINCTURE TONIC

This combination of herb tinctures can help stabilize symptoms that occur during perimenopause, the five to ten years before menstruation actually stops. Take this mixture to regulate off-kilter menstrual cycles or just to cool the occasional hot flush, says Virginia Frazer, a naturopathic doctor and licenced midwife.

Use a dosing syringe (available at most chemists) to accurately measure your doses. Take 5 millilitres of the blend two or three times a day, depending on the severity of your symptoms, says Dr Frazer. Tinctures tend to have a strong taste, so to make your herbal combo easier to swallow, add the measured amount to a half glass of water, tea or juice.

4 fl oz (120 ml)	**black cohosh**
2 fl oz (60 ml)	**partridgeberry (Mitchella repens, a Native American remedy, available by mail order or on the internet in the UK and Australia)**
2 fl oz (60 ml)	**motherwort**
1 fl oz (30 ml)	**agnus castus, or vitex**
1 fl oz (30 ml)	**wild yam**

Pour the black cohosh, partridgeberry, motherwort, agnus castus and wild yam into a glass mixing bowl, and set the empty bottles aside. Stir gently to blend, then use a small funnel to carefully rebottle your custom combination.

You might also consider including some iron-rich herbs in your diet. Try dandelion leaves, milk thistle seed, echinacea and peppermint. Eating them on the days you are bleeding heavily is best. You'll feel the effects within two weeks, and your next period won't bring heavy floods.

Yellow dock root. One problem with iron supplements is their tendency to cause constipation. That's why some popular herbal tonics include yellow dock root. While the herb is a source of iron, it also produces a gentle laxative effect. Thus, while it's contributing to your body's stores of iron, it can also help counter supplemental iron's constipating tendencies.

Yellow dock root also contains thiamin and vitamin C, which help the absorption of iron. It has 1 milligram of iron per 20-drop dose of alcohol tincture or three-teaspoon dose of vinegar tincture, says Susun

Weed. Either an alcohol or a vinegar tincture is fine, taken daily in tea or water. Iron is absorbed a little at a time, so she suggests taking yellow dock root throughout the day.

Vitamin C and bioflavonoids. Vitamin C can significantly increase iron absorption, so you should take it with your iron supplement. But the combination of vitamin C and bioflavonoids is better yet, according to Liz Collins, a naturopathic doctor.

If you're prone to excessive menstrual bleeding, it might be the result of fragile blood vessels. Vitamin C and bioflavonoids may strengthen those blood vessels, making them less susceptible to damage. In one study, for example, 14 out of 16 women who took supplements of 200 milligrams of vitamin C three times a day along with bioflavonoids found relief from heavy bleeding. Dr Collins recommends taking 500 to 1,000 milligrams of vitamin C three times a day, and 500 to 1,000 milligrams of bioflavonoids once a day.

Agnus castus. 'The single best herb for regulating the menstrual cycle is agnus castus,' says Dr Robert Rountree, a holistic doctor. When taken regularly, agnus castus regulates the timing of the menstrual cycle by acting on the pituitary gland, which in turn releases the hormones that regulate ovarian function. Recommended for a number of menstrual disorders by Germany's Commission E, which evaluates herbs for safety and effectiveness, agnus castus is now approved as a common treatment for menstrual irregularity. Take one or two 225-milligram capsules standardized for 0.5 per cent agnuside (an active component) every day. (This information should be on the bottle, or ask at the healthfood shop.) If you want to use the herb in a less medicinal way, grind the dried fruits and sprinkle them on your food for a peppery flavour.

Black cohosh. Among Native Americans, black cohosh was a widely used folk remedy for menstrual irregularities. As we mentioned earlier, black cohosh works as a mild oestrogen, like agnus castus. If your oestrogen levels are too low, plant oestrogens in the root, called isoflavones, pick up the slack and help regulate your cycle. Drink two to four dropperfuls of tincture in a little water or tea three times a day, or take two capsules of standardized extract daily, recommends Beverly Yates, a naturopathic doctor.

Cinnamon. Cinnamon is more than just a kitchen spice – it's been used medicinally for thousands of years. Ancient Chinese herbalists mention it as early as 2700 BC, and Chinese herbalists today still recommend it for keeping menstrual cycles regular and stemming heavy bleeding. If you are bleeding heavily, sip a cup of cinnamon infusion, chew a cinnamon stick, or take five to ten drops of tincture once or twice a day.

Angelica sinensis. As we mentioned earlier, Angelica sinensis is widely used in China and is commonly prescribed for menstrual irregularities. The phyto-oestrogens in this member of the carrot family help regulate and balance the menstrual cycle, especially if your periods are infrequent, says Dr Yates. Take ½ teaspoon of alcohol-based tincture in a glass of water up to four times a day. Women who are prone to heavy menstrual bleeding should avoid using this herb. Be especially cautious if you have uterine fibroids or endometriosis, as anything that might promote uterine bleeding could aggravate these conditions.

Lady's mantle. It's believed that this herb can prevent excessive bleeding when taken one to two weeks before menstruation. In a clinical study, lady's mantle tincture controlled menstrual flooding in virtually all of the 300 women who participated. When taken after flooding began, lady's mantle took three to five days to become effective. Experts suggest using five to ten drops of the fresh plant tincture three times a day for up to two weeks out of every month.

Vaginal Dryness

After menopause, your vaginal lining may begin to thin and dry out due to the lack of oestrogen. This can make sex painful or even undesirable. Surveys indicate that this happens in 8 to 25 per cent of postmenopausal women. While premenopausal women can generally lubricate in six to 20 seconds when aroused, it can take one to three minutes for a postmenopausal woman. Also, the thinning of the vaginal tissues makes the tissue more susceptible to irritation or trauma, which may provide a gateway for infection. Here are some ways to get relief.

Vitamin E. Take 400 international units of vitamin E each day. Recent research has paid little attention to the effects of vitamin E on vaginal dryness. But two studies done in the 1940s indicated that vitamin

E supplements can improve symptoms of vaginal atrophy, says Dr Michael Murray, a naturopathic doctor and health writer. These days, many doctors recommend vitamin E for vaginal dryness and other physical changes associated with menopause.

If you decide to try vitamin E, give yourself at least four weeks to see results. You can also use vitamin E topically. Simply pop open the capsule, put the oil on your finger and apply where it's needed. Do this twice a day or whenever you need relief.

Liquorice. Chew two tablets (a total of 380 milligrams) of deglycyrrhizinated liquorice root about 30 minutes before each meal. (Deglycyrrhizinated means that the compounds that elevate blood pressure have been removed; look for 'DGL' on the package.) Liquorice root targets vaginal dryness in two ways, according to Dr Helen Healy, a naturopathic doctor. For starters, the herb stimulates mucus production in your body and even increases the number of goblet cells (cells that manufacture mucus). Plus, liquorice root contains compounds that act as weak forms of oestrogen.

You can buy chewable tablets of deglycyrrhizinated liquorice root in healthfood shops. The tablets work so well, says Dr Healy, that you may find yourself having to blow your nose as you chew them. Forget about munching on liquorice sweets, though – they don't even contain real liquorice.

Panax ginseng. Take 100 milligrams of panax ginseng (sometimes called Asian ginseng), in the form of a standardized extract, once or twice a day. The active compounds in ginseng apparently have an oestrogen-like effect on vaginal tissue, helping it stay moist and supple. 'In traditional Chinese medicine, ginseng is often prescribed to women in their menopausal and postmenopausal years as a general tonic,' explains James E. Williams, a doctor of oriental medicine.

A standardized extract ensures that you are getting a consistent amount of the active compounds in ginseng – unlike most teas and herbal formulas, which contain very little of the compounds. Ask a medical professional who is knowledgeable about herbs to recommend a product to you, Dr Williams suggests. You can buy the extracts in healthfood shops. Just look for the words *standardized extract* on the label.

HERBAL FORMULAS COVER IT ALL

Many herbalists have their own special herbal tonics that they've used over the years to treat a spectrum of menopausal symptoms. Hot flushes plague you. Your sleep isn't very deep or very restful. Your moods are a touch volcanic. And the periods you're still having could be less, well, bloodily intense. Nothing you can't live with, but life could be a whole lot more comfortable without this cluster of annoyances. Here's what highly respected herbalists have to offer.

Keep in mind, though, that when it comes to menopause, each woman is different. One of these formulas may work better for you than another, so you may have to experiment to find the best blend. Remember, too, that herbs work slowly, so you might not feel any results at all for three weeks or so. Susun S. Weed, a herbalist and author of the *Wise Woman* series of herbal health books, urges women to begin with one herb if they are novices. If you take a lot of herbs at once and one of them doesn't agree with you, you won't know which one it is.

Try the menopause formula. Created by herbalists Cascade Anderson Geller and Valerie Perrine for the National College of Naturopathic Medicine in the US, 'this formula has helped women who are experiencing menopausal changes,' says Cascade, who is a consulting herbal practitioner and teacher of herbalism.

'If menopausal changes become increasingly intolerable, first consider improving your diet and lifestyle. Stick to a low-fat, high-fibre diet, drink lots of water and exercise for at least 30 minutes every other day,' she advises. 'If these changes don't bring relief, try my herbal formula. It has helped countless women ease the effects of menopause.' She adds, 'Get your doctor to monitor your progress. Tell her precisely what you're taking. Suggest that you may be able to take less oestrogen as a result. Ask her to monitor you closely as you ease off your oestrogen. Most GPs are more and more open-minded about herbs these days, and it's very important that you let your doctor know that you're taking herbs in the hope of taking less oestrogen.'

Menopause Formula

To make this formula, use the following herbal tinctures.

- 2   parts liquorice
- 2   parts dandelion root
- 1   part motherwort
- 1   part true unicorn root or false unicorn root
- 1   part wild yam

Using a funnel, pour the tinctures into a bottle large enough to hold 210 ml (about 7 fl oz). Add 1 to 3 dropperfuls of the tincture mixture to a little water, and drink two or three times a day three to five days a week.

Always take the lowest dose possible, and taper off as quickly as possible when symptoms diminish, Cascade advises.

Take one mixture for many ills. Agnus castus (chasteberry) helps balance hormones, motherwort has anti-anxiety and antispasmodic effects, and false unicorn has hormonal and digestive benefits, says Silena Heron, vice president of the Botanical Medicine Academy. Angelica sinensis, liquorice, black cohosh and alfalfa help enhance oestrogen activity. Black haw (or stagbush) reduces the spasticity that can promote hot flushes, and black cohosh relieves cramps. Sage decreases secretions, including sweat, which makes it useful for reducing both the frequency and severity of hot flushes. As a bonus, sage helps improve digestion, it's a source of zinc and it kills germs, too. Dr Heron includes St John's wort in her menopause formula because of its ability to ease pelvic complaints and depression.

'A woman benefits most from herbal therapy when the formula is adjusted to her specific needs,' says Dr Heron. 'But this basic formula has been so successful in relieving menopausal discomforts that many women return to my clinic just to have the prescription refilled.'

Dr Heron's Menopause Mixture

Dr Heron's formula is made by mixing the following herbal tinctures.

    2   parts agnus castus
    1   part motherwort
    1   part false unicorn root
    1   part Angelica sinensis
  1–2   parts sage
    1   part St John's wort
  1–2   parts black cohosh
  ½–1   part liquorice
  ½–1   part black haw (stagbush)
  ½–1   part alfalfa

Blend the herbal tinctures together in a bottle. Take half to one teaspoon three times a day on an empty stomach, on its own or mixed with a little water, advises Dr Heron.

HERBAL FORMULAS COVER IT ALL
— CONTINUED

Opt for a hormone helper. Rosemary Gladstar's Menopause Tincture will strengthen and tone the endocrine system, which is responsible for manufacturing your body's hormones. During menopause, the adrenal glands take on the role of producing oestrogen after the ovaries cease doing so, and they often need a boost during the transition, says herbalist Rosemary Gladstar, author of *The Family Herbal*. Each of the herbs in the formula helps revitalize the adrenal glands, she says. In addition, wild yam is known for its powerful effect on regulating hormone production, sarsaparilla* is said to aid body functioning as a whole, and black cohosh has traditionally been recommended for menopausal pains and discomfort.

Rosemary recommends using high-quality dried herbs that you tincture yourself, in good brandy or vodka. You can also make this formula from shop-bought tinctures. The formula will last you a very long time. Use the tonic consistently over an extended period of time to assure steady, long-lasting results, she adds.

Rosemary Gladstar's Menopause Tincture

- 2 parts wild yam
- 1 part sarsaparilla*
- 1 part black cohosh
- 2 parts Siberian ginseng
- 1 part Angelica sinensis
- 3 parts sage
- 3 parts liquorice
- 3 parts dandelion root

Black cohosh and Angelica sinensis. You'd be right if you guessed at this point that the all-around best herb for menopausal symptoms seems to be black cohosh. Along with its many other attributes, it also helps relieve vaginal dryness. You can combine black cohosh with Chinese angelica to get better results, if taking the herb individually doesn't relieve the dryness. Take 250 to 300 milligrams of black cohosh three times a day,

Mix the herbs together. Put four tablespoons of the mixture into a wide-mouth bottle and cover with 570 ml (1 pint) of good-quality brandy or vodka. Cover with a tight-fitting lid, place in a warm, shaded area, and let stand for four to six weeks. Shake daily to mix the herbs with the alcohol. After four to six weeks, strain into a clean bottle through a strainer lined with muslin. The recommended dose is ¼ teaspoon three times a day for three months or longer. Rosemary suggests that you dilute the tincture in water, juice or decaffeinated or herbal tea before drinking.

*If you have trouble finding sarsaparilla (also known as wild liquorice) in your local healthfood shop, you will be able to find it on the internet, or buy it through mail order.

To prevent irritability, avoid consuming caffeine and other stimulants while using ginseng.

Sip some menopause tea. If you prefer drinking tea, rather than taking an alcohol-based tincture, try this blend, created by herbalist Amanda McQuade Crawford, author of the *Herbal Menopause Book*. Use high-quality dried herbs. All quantities are dry weight, not liquid.

Amanda's Menopause Tea

90 g (3 oz)	agnus castus
60 g (2 oz)	Angelica sinensis
30 g (1 oz)	Siberian ginseng or liquorice
60 g (2 oz)	St John's wort
60 g (2 oz)	horsetail
90 g (3 oz)	motherwort
1	organic orange, or lemon rind (for flavour)

Mix the herbs together well. Infuse 30 g (1 oz) of herbal blend in 1.1 litres (2 pints) of boiling water, cover and steep for 20 minutes, then strain. Amanda recommends that you drink one large glass three times a day.

says Dr Collins. If you combine it with Chinese angelica, take up to 4,000 milligrams of each per day for up to six months. Some women start with 4,000 milligrams per day and then, once their symptoms are under control, decrease the dose slowly to find the minimum dose that maintains control.

Mood Swings

In menopause, you can be merry one moment and maniacal the next – without rhyme nor reason, it seems. According to one theory, the hormonal downdrafts and upsurges of menopause trigger mood swings in an unpredictable and sometimes indirect way. Here's how to take the 'menace' out of menopause.

Calcium. Boosting your calcium intake may give relief from irritability. In a five-and-a-half-month study at the Grand Forks Human Nutrition Research Center of the US Department of Agriculture, women who were given 1,300 milligrams of calcium daily reported far fewer woes than those who got 600 milligrams daily. Nine of the ten women had fewer mood changes, such as irritability and depression, says Dr James G. Penland, a research psychologist at the Center. Taking calcium supplements can also lead to less difficulty concentrating. In one of the largest studies of calcium for PMS, researchers found that women taking 1,200 milligrams of calcium daily for three menstrual cycles experienced a more positive mood. Researchers suspect that calcium relieves PMS by easing depression, but they have not yet discovered how.

Magnesium and vitamin B_6. These nutrients help assure a healthy supply of serotonin and dopamine, two mood-regulating neurotransmitters. Women can supplement their diets with 350 milligrams of magnesium and 100 milligrams of vitamin B_6, says Dr George J. Kallins, an assistant clinical professor of obstetrics and gynaecology in California. However, you should get your dose of B_6 through a multivitamin or B complex supplement, he says. The B vitamins work together, which means that supplemental B_6 won't be helpful unless you also have adequate amounts of the other B vitamins.

Pantothenic acid. Some studies indicate that many people in the West aren't getting enough of this B vitamin. The UK RNI is 6 milligrams; Australia and New Zealand have no recommended recommended daily intake. Studies show, however, that many of us get only about half of what we need from our diets. Deficiencies have been known to produce depression and fatigue. Taking 500 milligrams a day may bolster your mood, says Dr Willow Moore, a chiropractor and naturopathic doctor. Pantothenic acid is sometimes labelled as vitamin B$_5$. (Other forms include calcium pantothenate and pantethine.)

Black cohosh. Once again, black cohosh is voted the herb most likely to succeed by natural practitioners. German physicians have been recommending it since the 1940s for hormone disturbances. Herbalists suggest taking half to one millilitre of tincture two to four times daily for relief of hormone-related mood swings.

Chamomile. 'I've had high-powered executives say, "My doctor wants to put me on Xanax [an anti-anxiety prescription medication]",' says Patricia Howell, a professional member of the American Herbalists Guild (AHG). 'Instead, I put them on chamomile tea, and they've told me that they felt their lives were theirs again.'

But the chamomile tea that Howell recommends is much stronger than the average brew. To make this chamomile infusion, put 60–90 g (2–3 oz) of dried chamomile flowers in a jar and cover it with freshly boiled water. Let it steep overnight. Then strain out the herb and drink about 60 ml of

SUPER SUPPLEMENT CHECKLIST No. 3

If you're concerned about heart disease, try these supplements. As you can see, the list is extensive, so make sure you read the descriptions, choose the ones you think are right for you, and check with your doctor before beginning a supplement programme.

- ☐ Vitamin E
- ☐ Fat-soluble vitamin C
- ☐ Folic acid
- ☐ Vitamin B$_{12}$
- ☐ Vitamin B$_6$
- ☐ Niacin
- ☐ Fish oils
- ☐ Coenzyme Q$_{10}$
- ☐ Aspirin
- ☐ Fibre
- ☐ Black tea
- ☐ Amino acids
- ☐ Garlic supplements
- ☐ Guggul (an Indian herb)
- ☐ Magnesium
- ☐ Potassium
- ☐ Calcium
- ☐ Ginger
- ☐ Fenugreek
- ☐ Turmeric
- ☐ Dandelion root

VITAMIN E: NATURAL SUPPLEMENTS ARE TWICE AS GOOD

A generation ago, vitamin C topped the hit parade of vitamins, says Dr Maret Traber, associate professor in the department of nutrition and food management at Oregon State University. These days vitamin E gets all the attention.

Dr Traber ought to know: she's principal investigator for the Linus Pauling Institute, and she rates vitamin E an 'E for excellent' when it comes to helping to prevent heart disease and cancer. It can also clear the lungs of air pollutants – *if* you get enough vitamin E, that is.

As premier member of a class of nutrients known as antioxidants, vitamin E protects your body against destructive oxygen molecules in your body by taking a spare electron from the harmful 'free radicals' inside your cells. In your lungs, vitamin E protects you against nitrogen dioxide, ozone and other pollutants that can oxidize cells in your lungs, allowing you to breathe more easily.

The UK RNA and the Australian RDI for vitamin E is 10 milligrams or 15 International Units (IU), but medical experts who have studied the benefits of E recommend 100 to 200 IU a day – more than you can realistically expect to get from even the richest dietary sources, so make sure you take a supplement. You'd have to eat 900 g (2 lb) of peanuts or 7 kg (16 lb) of boiled spinach to get 100 IU.

this fairly strong infusion, hot or cold, as needed for anxiety and accompanying digestive upset.

'It is a very strong preparation and can be taken as often as needed,' she says. 'It can be diluted with hot water to make a weaker tea.' (For an easier method, use two or three chamomile tea bags rather than the loose herb.)

Skullcap. Skullcap tincture strengthens the nerves, eases oversensitivity, and helps promote deep, sound sleep, says Susun Weed. She uses four to eight drops of the tincture mornings and evenings when she's feeling 'fried, stressed-out, wired, or just wound up'. (Do not confuse it with Chinese skullcap, though, which has entirely different properties.)

Agnus castus. Take five to 15 drops of agnus castus tincture, mixed with a few fluid ounces (about 75 ml) of water, three times a day. Agnus castus is commonly prescribed in European countries for PMS. The herb

'Even in the healthiest of diets, we don't get enough vitamin E,' says Dr Traber. 'So supplements are important.'

Which vitamin E supplements are better, natural or synthetic? Several studies support the use of vitamin E in its natural form, d-alpha tocopherol, over its synthetic form, dl-alpha tocopherol. (Natural vitamin E supplements start with the letter 'd', such as 'd-alpha tocopherol'. Synthetic vitamin E products start with the letters 'dl'.) For one thing, it's twice as active – you'd need 400 IU of synthetic vitamin E to equal 200 IU of natural vitamin E. But your body also retains natural vitamin E three times as long as the synthetic, which means it can build up and maintain higher levels of protection.

Foods contain not one but eight types of vitamin E molecules – alpha, beta, gamma and delta tocopherols, and alpha, beta, gamma and delta tocotrienols. So experts say that even if you rely partially on supplements, you should aim to include good sources of vitamin E in your diet: soya bean and corn oils and avocados, peanut butter, wheat germ and sunflower seeds.

Large doses of vitamin E may increase the risk of bleeding problems and lead to strokes. So before taking vitamin E supplements, check with your doctor, especially if you have high blood pressure, if you smoke, if you have had a stroke or if there is a history of stroke in your family, or if you take blood thinners (anticoagulants) or regular doses of aspirin for a heart condition.

appears to work through the pituitary, your body's master gland, to help re-establish hormonal balance, says Dr Daniel Mowrey, in his book *Herbal Tonic Therapies*. If you prefer to take vitex, which is the fruit of the chaste-tree, try taking two 500-milligram tablets twice a day for a few months to see if it helps. If it does, you should keep taking it. In a German study, women who took vitex and then gave it up had a return of symptoms within three months.

Healing the Heart

By now, we all know that once a woman enters menopause, her oestrogen production begins to slow down. A woman's risk of heart disease rises every year after menopause. Fortunately, there are many ways to minimize and even reverse any existing damage by living a heart-friendly lifestyle that includes managing high blood pressure and high cholesterol through a balanced diet. Women with a nutritious diet will get most of the nutrients that they need for long-term heart health, but herbs and supplements can provide some extra insurance.

Vitamin E. Studies have shown that women who take vitamin E supplements reduce their risk of heart attack by up to 41 per cent. Vitamin E may help prevent heart disease in several ways. Its most important role may be helping to prevent ravages of free radicals – harmful oxygen molecules your body produces that damage tissues throughout the body. These molecules cause cholesterol to cling to artery walls and clog them up. Vitamin E can help prevent the cholesterol buildup by getting rid of free radicals before they do any damage. Slowing this oxidation process may limit cholesterol's propensity to clog up arteries. Vitamin E may also help prevent platelets from aggregating along the blood vessel walls, which promotes blood clotting.

Many doctors advise women to take 100 to 400 IU vitamin E daily. At the same time, it's helpful to take a multivitamin that also contains vitamin C, another antioxidant that 'recharges' vitamin E in the body and increases its effectiveness.

Fat-soluble vitamin C. Vitamin C keeps our arterial walls from thinning as we age, says Dr Maria Sulindro, president and founder of eAntiAging.com, an internet organization that provides scientific information about anti-ageing approaches. When the walls thin, they have a tendency to crack and leak. This process causes inflammation, enabling the undesirable, LDL cholesterol to accumulate along the inner walls of the coronary arteries.

The most common form of vitamin C, ascorbic acid, is water-soluble and won't reach the vascular wall, says Dr Sulindro. 'Instead, take 1,000 to 2,000 milligrams of fat-soluble vitamin C, ascorbyl palmitate. This form stays in the body longer, having more chance to get to the arterial wall,' she says. (If you are on a cholesterol-lowering drug, check with your doctor before taking supplemental vitamin C.)

Even in people with healthy intakes of vitamin C, additional vitamin C seems to help increase HDL levels. In one study at the Jean Mayer

USDA Human Nutrition Research Center on Aging, men and women with low blood levels of vitamin C who took 1,000 milligrams of supplemental vitamin C a day for eight months averaged a 7 per cent increase in their HDL readings.

Folic acid. Unless you eat fortified breakfast cereals, you'd have to eat the equivalent of more than 285 g (10 oz) of Cos lettuce daily to meet the daily requirement of folic acid. Take 800 micrograms to help lower your cholesterol, says Dr Stephen T. Sinatra, a cardiologist.

B vitamins. This family of vitamins is heart-friendly because they help your body chew up homocysteine, a substance that you can easily do without. Homocysteine is an amino acid by-product that can damage arteries. It creates rough spots on artery walls, and those roughened areas can pick up fatty deposits that harden into artery-clogging plaque. Taking the vitamins we recommend below can help keep your artery walls smooth.

Vitamin B_{12}. Your options for getting this vitamin through your diet are limited. It is found in red meat, but our hearts can do without the artery-clogging fats that come with the whole package. Take 20 micrograms of vitamin B_{12}, recommends Dr Sinatra.

Vitamin B_6. Even if your homocysteine levels are low, a deficiency of vitamin B_6 will still put you at risk for heart disease. You need this nutrient to help your body use protein, fats and carbohydrates properly. B_6 also helps convert the amino acid tryptophan into another essential B vitamin, niacin. Dr Sinatra recommends taking 20 milligrams of B_6.

Niacin. In large doses, niacin raises HDL, the good cholesterol, and can lower LDL cholesterol, HDL's evil twin. It also lowers fibrinogen, a blood protein that causes clot formation. However, niacin is not universally effective, and it is also not a supplement you can safely take with cholesterol-lowering drugs. You need to talk to your doctor before taking niacin, to make sure it's right for you.

Fish oils. If you are at risk for heart disease, your doctor has probably told you to cut back on saturated fats, including animal fat, butter and the kind that's in many cakes, biscuits and pastries. Instead of those unhealthy fats, get more essential fatty acids, says Dr Decker Weiss, a naturopathic doctor. Omega-3 and omega-6 fatty acids change your body chemistry so that you produce less of the harmful prostaglandins, hormonelike substances that can narrow the arteries, cause excessive blood clotting and hike up blood pressure. 'I recommend 1,000 to 3,000 milligrams a day of a mixture of these two essential fatty acids,' he says.

Coenzyme Q_{10}. This nutrient boosts the heart's pumping ability by improving energy supplies to the heart muscle cells, so it helps the heart to pump more efficiently with less effort. It may also help your liver withstand the toxicity of statin drugs, and it reduces their side-effects, such as liver problems and muscle aches. However, a number of medicines, including antidepressants and cholesterol-lowering drugs, can deplete coenzyme Q_{10} from your body. As for how much to take, Dr Weiss suggests a dosage ranging from 30 to 50 milligrams a day.

Aspirin. Those humble little aspirins you thought were good only to dull your headaches are such valuable weapons against heart attacks that even some doctors are popping them daily. And when you team up aspirin with another common item on your shelf – vitamin E – you've got an anti-heart attack combo that's about as safe, cheap and simple as it is effective.

Aspirin helps prevent heart attacks by discouraging blood cells known as platelets from sticking together. This is great for women because heart attacks experienced by women are likelier to be caused by blood clots than by blocked arteries, which usually trigger heart attacks in men.

How much aspirin will your doctor recommend? It depends.

If you've been diagnosed with coronary heart disease but have not had a heart attack. You might reduce your chances of a heart attack by a third by taking aspirin regularly. 'Women with coronary disease should be taking an aspirin every day,' says Dr Nanette Wenger, professor of medicine and head of cardiology at a large hospital.

If you've had a heart attack. Taking anything from a junior aspirin (80 milligrams) to one adult aspirin (325 milligrams) daily may prevent another one.

If you're having a heart attack. Taking a 325-milligram aspirin straight away may improve your survival chances by 25 per cent. Yale researchers found that one reason top hospitals save more heart attack patients may be that they're more forthcoming with the aspirin.

If you don't have coronary heart disease but do have risk factors such as diabetes or high cholesterol. Follow your doctor's recommendation. A woman without heart disease or without multiple risk factors runs such a low risk of heart attack that it's not worth risking minor or unlikely complications of taking aspirin, like stomach irritation, bleeding and, rarely, haemorrhagic stroke.

Fibre. Fibre is routinely prescribed for people concerned about heart disease because it binds with bile, which is secreted by your liver into the small intestine, and escorts it from your body. That means fats won't be reabsorbed into your system.

There is also some evidence that fibre can help reduce high blood pressure. In a study of more than 40,000 nurses whose lifestyles and diet patterns were followed for four years, researchers discovered that those who got the highest amounts of fibre were least likely to develop high blood pressure.

In another study, with animals whose blood pressures had been elevated by high-fat diets, switching to a low-fat diet and taking fibre supplements reduced blood pressure by ten to 15 points.

Of the two kinds of fibre – soluble and insoluble – it's the soluble type that is more important for reducing cholesterol and lowering blood pressure. This fibre is found in fruit, beans and oats. If you want additional fibre, look for a supplement that contains mixed soluble fibres, such as psyllium, oat bran, gums and pectin.

Black tea. If you're at risk for a heart attack, your doctor may prescribe daily aspirin and vitamin E supplements. If so, consider washing them down with tea.

When researchers considered the coffee- and tea-drinking habits of several hundred men and women, people who drank tea regularly had about half the heart attack risk of those who didn't drink tea. (Coffee consumption had no effect on the risk of heart attacks.) The tea in question is black tea. It's rich in flavonoids, natural antioxidants that researchers suspect may account for tea's apparent heart benefits. Moderate tea drinking – one or two cups a day – will do you no harm, and may do your heart a world of good, says Dr Howard Sesso, the Harvard Medical School epidemiologist who led the study.

GINGER-GARLIC SUPER SOUP

Both ginger and garlic are great for boosting the immune system, says Dr Mary Bove, a naturopathic doctor. Here's Dr Bove's recipe for protecting and strengthening your immunity. (The mung bean sprouts are added for extra doses of folate, potassium and magnesium for overall good health – not to mention a little added texture!)

1 l (1³/₄ pt)	**chicken or vegetable stock**
60 g (2 oz)	**finely chopped fresh garlic**
60 g (2 oz)	**finely sliced fresh ginger**
60 g (2 oz)	**mung bean sprouts***

Place the stock in a large saucepan and warm over medium-high heat. In a medium saucepan, sauté the garlic and ginger for three or four minutes, or until soft. Add to the stock. Stir in the sprouts and simmer for two or three minutes, or until heated through. Enjoy!

* If you can't get the sprouts at your local supermarket, buy the dried beans and grow your own.

Amino acids. The amino acids L-lysine and L–proline can help clear the LDL cholesterol that clogs blood circulation. 'This clogging represents half of all deaths of heart disease patients,' says Dr Sulindro. Get your doctor's approval before taking these amino acids.

Garlic supplements. The benefits of garlic are well-known, so if you are a garlic fan, go ahead and eat your fill. (Try our Ginger-garlic Super Soup if you want a delicious dose of 'medicine' for high cholesterol and blood pressure.) For many people, however, consistently eating five or more garlic cloves a day to lower cholesterol is more than they can relish. If you're among the lukewarm fans of whole garlic, the capsules are worth a try before you take cholesterol-lowering drugs.

Look for dried garlic powder preparation in enteric-coated tablets or capsules. These are designed to pass through the stomach and then degrade in the alkaline environment of the intestine, where the beneficial conversion of one compound, alliin, into the active ingredient, allicin, takes place. In studies it's been found that with supplements, people can lower total cholesterol by 10 to 12 per cent, and LDL and triglycerides by about 15 per cent. HDL levels usually increased by about 10 per cent. For those results, you'll need a preparation that provides a daily dose of at least 10 milligrams of alliin, or a total allicin potential of 4,000 micrograms. You'll probably need to allow one to three months before you begin seeing a change in your cholesterol levels.

Guggul. Guggul is a gum resin loosely related to myrrh. The herb has come into the spotlight for its ability to lower cholesterol. Guggul helps the liver create more receptors for LDL, which enables the liver to 'catch' more LDL from the blood and excrete it. Look for products that offer it in standardized form. The recommended standardized dosage is 25 milligrams three times a day. A person should take guggul until lipid levels normalize, and then should reduce the dose to 25 milligrams once a day.

Magnesium. If you have high blood pressure (consistently higher than 140/90), you may be low in magnesium. Those who find that salt raises their blood pressure may be low in this mineral, as well as in potassium, calcium and others. Magnesium helps to relax the smooth muscles in the blood vessels, which allows them to dilate.

If you are taking a diuretic for blood pressure control, it may be depleting your magnesium supply. The diuretic may actually stop working after six months if your magnesium stores are low. 'Supplemental magnesium sometimes make the diuretic more effective again,' says Dr Weiss. It's safe for most people to use up to 350 milligrams a day, he says. The preferred forms are magnesium orotate and magnesium glycinate.

Potassium. Potassium affects blood volume because it helps you excrete sodium, says Dr David B. Young, a professor of physiology and biophysics. When you excrete sodium, you also excrete water, which reduces blood volume and in turn reduces blood pressure. The safest way to get potassium is from foods, he says. Baked potatoes, prune juice, avocados and fat-free yoghurt contain plentiful amounts of this mineral. In supplement form, a prescription is needed for dosages higher than 99 milligrams per tablet. If you are taking a diuretic for high blood pressure, you may need supplemental potassium, Dr Young says. In this case, your doctor will monitor your blood levels.

Calcium. Like magnesium and potassium, calcium has a direct effect on blood volume or influences the ability of blood vessels to relax. The UK RNI for calcium is 700 mg, while the Australian RDI is 800 mg, an amount that many of us fail to consume in our daily diets. Even if you're not getting the recommended amount, though, if you already have high blood pressure, you should check with your doctor before taking supplemental calcium, Dr Weiss says. 'I don't normally recommend it for high blood pressure, unless I'm seeing an older woman who also has osteoporosis, because too much calcium can interfere with magnesium's muscle-relaxing ability.'

Ginger. Ginger gives you a double bonus of protection because it temporarily lowers elevated blood pressure and reduces LDL while raising HDL levels. In addition, ginger can help ward off strokes and heart attacks because it keeps platelets from aggregating.

Take one capsule of ginger, equivalent to 500 milligrams, three times a day. Then take less or more depending on what your lipid profile looks like after eight weeks. Ginger remains medicinally potent when you cook with it, and crystallized ginger and pickled ginger (the kind you get in Japanese restaurants) are also effective *and* tasty. (For a delicious way to pamper your heart, try the Ginger-garlic Super Soup recipe on page 114.)

Fenugreek. Consume one to two tablespoons of ground fenugreek seeds three or four times a day, suggests Dr Mary Bove, a naturopathic doctor and director of the Brattleboro Naturopathic Clinic. In one study, at the National Institute of Nutrition in India, people who ingested roughly 100 g (3½ oz) of the herb every day for 20 days cut their LDL levels by one-third. Even better, their HDL levels remained unchanged.

Fenugreek has a bittersweet liquorice taste. Try sprinkling some of the ground seeds on food. Or make a tea by steeping a fenugreek tea bag (available at healthfood shops) or 1 teaspoon of ground seeds in a mugful of freshly boiled water. If the taste of fenugreek doesn't appeal to you, take one or two 580-milligram capsules of the herb three or four times a day.

Turmeric. Researchers in India – where turmeric is a staple ingredient – have found that the herb enhances your body's ability to process cholesterol. As an alternative to using ground turmeric in your cooking, take 150 milligrams of the herb in capsule form three times a day, suggests Dr Bove. Turmeric capsules are available at most healthfood shops.

Dandelion root. Natural healers often concentrate on the connection between blood cholesterol and your liver. 'A neglected liver can really elevate cholesterol,' says Dr Pamela Sky Jeanne, a naturopathic family doctor. 'Your digestive system may not be eliminating the cholesterol, or your liver may be overproducing it.' That's where dandelion can help. Although there's no direct evidence linking dandelion and reduced cholesterol levels, there's no doubt that it's a great herb for your liver, according to naturopathic doctors. It's easy to find, but make sure the tincture is made from the root, says Dr Jeanne.

Use the bottle's dropper to fill a teaspoon, put the tincture in a small amount of water, and drink it down. It's best to take dandelion for about two months and then stop for about two weeks, says Dr Jeanne. You can then take it for another two months and continue the cycle until your cholesterol is lowered.

Some doctors prescribe dandelion as a natural potassium-sparing diuretic for high blood pressure, but the dosage depends on your blood pressure. If you have high blood pressure, see your doctor first before trying dandelion.

Combating Cancer

For many of us, *cancer* is one of the scariest words in the English language. And it's one we never want to hear applied to us. Because menopause increases your risk of hormone-related cancers such as endometrial and breast cancers (we'll tell you why in a minute), it makes sense to do everything you can to prevent them. And supplements can help. Research has shown that a host of supplements have anti-cancer properties. Read on to find out what they are and how to take them.

Endometrial Cancer

Endometrial cancer – cancer of the lining of the uterus – is the most common reproductive cancer in women. And menopause increases your risk. With low levels of oestrogen and progesterone, the endometrium doesn't slough off as it did during menstruation. The endometrial cells are still there, and with maturity they become more vulnerable to cancer.

SUPER SUPPLEMENT CHECKLIST No. 4

Add these supplements to your diet if you're concerned about cancer. They've been shown to have anti-cancer properties. Fortunately, many of them help with other menopause-related conditions as well!

☐ Vitamin E as oil (not dry)   ☐ Calcium
☐ Water-soluble vitamin C   ☐ Green tea
☐ Bioflavonoids   ☐ Garlic
☐ Carotenoids   ☐ Fibre
☐ Selenium   ☐ Flaxseed (Linseed)
☐ Folic acid

Oestrogen therapy increases the risk because taking too much oestrogen gets the endometrium growing again. The more growth and the more cells there are, the higher the likelihood that one cell will turn cancerous. That's why most hormone replacement therapy (HRT) includes progestin (a synthetic form of progesterone) with the oestrogen. Progesterone helps protect against endometrial cancer by 'calming down' the oestrogen-stimulated cells.

Breast Cancer

Rates of breast cancer are highest in the Western world. Other than skin cancer, it is the most common form of malignancy diagnosed among women in the UK: 33,000 women are diagnosed with breast cancer every year, and each year 14,000 women die of the disease. In Australia, breast cancer is the most common cause of cancer-related death in women. Nationally, more than 7,500 women are diagnosed with breast cancer each year and approximately 2,500 die of it. These figures are much the same per capita in New Zealand, and in South Africa, the incidence is rising by 2 per cent per year. Only lung cancer is more lethal. Since 1973, the number of breast cancers diagnosed has increased about 2 per cent annually, although much of that increase is the result of better methods of detection.

Doctors aren't certain what makes the breast so susceptible to cancer, but a number of factors are known to increase a woman's risk of developing the disease, including age and oestrogen exposure.

Age. A woman's risk of breast cancer increases gradually as she gets older. It is rarely diagnosed in women under the age of 35, but all women aged 40 and over are at increased risk. Most cases occur in women over 50, and the risk is particularly high among women over the age of 60.

Oestrogen exposure. Women who experience menopause after age 55, or who have taken hormone replacement therapy for a number of years, may be at a higher risk for breast cancer. And the longer you are exposed to oestrogen, the likelier you are to develop it.

Risk factors are important, but paying too much attention to them may be misleading, as the odds that any one of them will trigger breast cancer are less than 1 per cent, says Dr Deborah Capko, a breast surgeon and associate medical director of the Institute for Breast Care in the US. In fact, many women with known risk factors do not get breast cancer. And many women who have no factors develop the disease. Doctors are hard-pressed to explain this paradox. That is why diligence is critical.

There are no known absolute ways to prevent breast cancer, but some supplements and herbs may help reduce your risk.

Antioxidants. Researchers speculate that up to 30 per cent of cancers are affected simply by what we eat. Vegetables and fruit supply your body with an armoury of antioxidants. Getting the requisite five or more servings a day of fruit and vegetables is the first step in defending yourself against cancer. But while prevention may start at your plate, you can go even further with specific antioxidant supplements known for their anti-cancer actions, says Dr Keith Berndtson, an expert in integrative medicine. In addition to a healthy diet, he says, 'I'd stick to a high-potency multiple vitamin tablet with additional antioxidants for cancer prevention.'

Vitamins E and C. Two of the most important antioxidants are also the most well-known – vitamin E and vitamin C. These two are favourites when it comes to improving overall health, and for cancer prevention, they seem to be all-stars.

Oily vitamin E is hard to get in abundance from dietary sources alone. Supplemental amounts from 400 to 800 international units (IU) a day are recommended by Dr W. John Diamond, medical director of the Triad

Medical Center, and co-author of *An Alternative Medicine Definitive Guide to Cancer.*

Water-soluble vitamin C is relatively easy to find in foods. Although the UK RNI for C is only 40 milligrams, the same as it is in Australia and New Zealand, Dr Diamond suggests much more for the prevention and treatment of cancer. He recommends between 1,000 and 8,000 milligrams in divided doses throughout the day.

Bioflavonoids. Hidden inside vegetables, fruit, flowers, herbs and grains are compounds commonly known as bioflavonoids. Researchers regard them as powerful antioxidants because they provide protection against free radicals. These compounds may have anti-cancer properties. Bioflavonoids are widely available in supplements as quercetin, rutin or hesperidin. You'll also see supplements called proanthocyanidins, or PCOs, which are derived primarily from red wines and grapeseed extracts. These multi-talented substances may have remarkable effects, one of which could be their ability to convert malignant cells into normal cells.

While the many benefits of bioflavonoids are being explored, experts are still trying to decide whether most of us can benefit from supplementation. Some say that we get all the bioflavonoids we need from our diets and that supplementing provides no additional benefits. Others argue that supplements provide extra protection and help fill the gaps when our diets are lacking. If you decide you would like to supplement your diet with bioflavonoids, talk to your doctor first before you do.

Carotenoids. Nutrition researchers have distinguished another group of antioxidants, called carotenoids. These substances are also associated with a reduced risk of cancer. In most studies, however, researchers studied the effects of carotenoid-rich foods rather than supplements. The most studied has been beta-carotene. In early studies, researchers found that the group of people who got the largest amount of this nutrient from foods also had substantially fewer cancers. Beta-carotene was hailed as the newest antioxidant vitamin, able to protect not only the outsides of cells against free radicals, but also the insides, providing a stronger defence against damage.

When researchers started studying supplements of beta-carotene, however, they observed that the benefits didn't apply to everyone who upped their consumption. For smokers, beta-carotene might have a negative

VITAMIN C: YOUR ALL-DAY POLLUTION SHIELD

Back at school, we all learned that scientists discovered our need for vitamin C by accident, when British sailors deprived of fresh fruit and vegetables developed scurvy. Today we need more vitamin C than ever. Vitamin C naturally battles toxins, fortifying us against cigarette smoke, exhaust fumes, smog and other pollutants that – except for the occasional volcanic eruption – didn't exist back in the past.

'Smokers need more vitamin C than non-smokers because what they are inhaling is essentially highly polluted air,' says Dr Robert A. Jacob, a research chemist for the USDA Western Human Nutrition Research Center.

Even if you don't live in a smog capital like London or spend hours in bumper-to-bumper traffic, you need vitamin C. This water-soluble antioxidant helps to detoxify your system by activating glutathione, a sulphurlike antioxidant, inside the body. Antioxidants eliminate cell-damaging molecules known as free radicals.

'Vitamin C not only neutralizes free radicals by itself but works with glutathione to eliminate other potential toxins you might take in through food or drugs,' says Dr Jacob. Vitamin C also helps your immune system protect you against infections and chronic illnesses.

Kilo for kilo, women need less vitamin C than men. That's because vitamin C is used by muscle, not fat, and because women typically have less muscle mass, we need less vitamin C to derive the same benefits. However, Dr Jacob recommends that women and men both get at least 60 milligrams of vitamin C a day, and smokers 100 milligrams a day. Your body can absorb only so much vitamin C at a time. So if you take supplements, try to spread out your vitamin C supplements throughout the day.

effect. This has led experts to be wary of recommending supplemental beta-carotene to everyone. True, a nutrient that poses a risk to smokers might be beneficial rather than harmful to non-smokers. Smokers are already at high risk of cancer, and perhaps because of that, they react differently to beta-carotene than do non-smokers. Researchers are wondering, though, whether it might be harmful to take beta-carotene in isolation from the rest of the carotenoids, and with that question still hanging, a beta–carotene supplement can't be recommended as an across-the-board preventive. The moderate doses of carotenoids that come from foods, however, continue to show substantial anti-cancer promise.

If you want to add carotenoids to your diet, you might try a supplement called mixed carotenoids, says Dr Berndtson. Look for one that supplies beta–carotene as well as the carotenoids gamma–carotene, lycopene, lutein and zeaxanthin, he advises.

Selenium. Supplementing your diet with a small amount of the trace mineral selenium may make a huge dent in your cancer risk. A ten-year study found that men and women who took selenium supplements had a 37 per cent lower incidence of cancer than those who took a placebo. The supplements appeared to have a significant impact on colon cancer, cutting incidence of the disease by 58 per cent, and lung cancer, cutting incidence by 46 per cent. It's possible that selenium may encourage abnormal cells and small, undetected tumours to self-destruct before they can cause trouble. The people who participated in the study took 200 micrograms daily. Check with your doctor, however, before you start taking this much.

Folic acid. Cancer can be the result of an accumulation of damage to DNA over time. Smoking, exposure to harmful chemicals, frequent exposure to x-rays and certain viruses can damage a cell's genetic material. Add the injury of folic acid shortage to any one of these insults, and 'you are turning up the speed of damage severalfold,' explains Dr Patrick Stover, assistant professor of nutritional biochemistry and cell biology at Cornell University.

In several studies, folic acid deficiency has been strongly linked to DNA damage. In one, researchers at the University of California found that even a mild deficiency caused a large increase in the amount of damaged DNA. Other studies have shown a link between folic acid deficiency and dysplasia (abnormal, precancerous cells) in the cervix, colon and lungs.

Most people get about 200 micrograms of folate a day, about half the UK RNI and the Australian and New Zealand RDI. With folic acid–fortified foods, such as breads and breakfast cereals, now on the market, daily intake could increase on average to about 300 micrograms a day, leaving a 100-microgram deficit. Most over-the-counter multivitamins contain 400 micrograms, and a few super-potency vitamins provide 800 micrograms. You should never take more than 1,000 micrograms without checking with your doctor first.

Calcium. This mineral is found in broccoli, grapefruit, brussels sprouts, apples and, of course, milk. But you don't have to drink three glasses of milk a day if you don't want to. In its supplement form, calcium is a real powerhouse against cancer. 'It has been found to fight cancers of the skin, breasts, ovaries, lungs and bones,' says Dr Sulindro. It's also being studied as a way to prevent breast cancer in high-risk women.

Calcium works in the liver to chemically change cancer-causing substances so they pass quickly through the body without doing any harm. Dosage recommendations are anywhere from 200 to 2,000 milligrams daily, says Dr Sulindro, so check with your doctor. For better absorption, spread your doses out over the day, and take no more than 500 milligrams at once. If you use calcium citrate, lactate or gluconate, you can take it between meals without absorption problems, and it won't interfere with iron and other trace minerals. All other forms of supplemental calcium are best absorbed when taken with food.

Green tea. The traditional pale green brew that accompanies Japanese food appears to have potent anti-cancer properties, according to Dr Jerzy Jankun, a cancer researcher and associate professor of urology.

Green tea contains a substance called epigallocathechin-3 gallate (EGCG). Dr Jankun's research shows that EGCG inhibits urokinase, an enzyme that allows tumours to grow and spread. 'By inhibiting urokinase, those processes *could* be stopped,' says Dr Jankun. 'EGCG has been known to possess other anti-cancer activity, but inhibition of urokinase seems to be the most important factor.'

How much green tea should you sip? You can follow the lead from the East: Asian tea lovers commonly drink up to ten cups a day. While this may seem like a lot, research suggests that consuming such a large quantity may be necessary to reap green tea's anti-cancer benefits. If you prefer your protection in capsules rather than cups, green tea extract is available in supplement form, says Dr Jankun. Sometimes an equivalent in cups will be noted on the label, or the label will give the concentration of green tea in milligrams. Since potencies are different, follow the directions on the label. Most brands advise taking one or two capsules two or three times a day.

Garlic. Research suggests that garlic and other members of the onion family can cut your odds of developing cancer. In once study, women who ate garlic at least once a week cut their colon cancer risks by one-third, compared with women who never ate the stuff. If you avoid fresh garlic because you don't like it or it doesn't agree with you, look for dried garlic powder preparation in enteric-coated tablets or capsules. Follow the directions on the label.

Fibre. Women whose diets include lots of fibrous foods – such as fruit, vegetables and wholewheat cereals and breads – may have fewer breast, colon and rectal cancers than those who don't eat those foods. Fibre reduces the amount of oestrogen in the blood. Oestrogen possibly alters cell structure and promotes breast cancer. In addition, fibre helps speed stool through your body, reducing the exposure of your digestive tract to carcinogens.

Fibre may also help prevent other cancers. In a study of 399 women with endometrial cancer and 296 disease-free women, researchers found that women who ate more than two servings of high-fibre breads and cereals a day had 40 per cent less risk of developing endometrial cancer.

If you aren't getting the 20 to 30 grams of fibre a day recommended by most cancer research groups, then consider taking a fibre supplement, like Metamucil.

Flaxseed (Linseed). Flaxseed is an incredibly rich source of a group of compounds called lignans. While many plant foods also contain lignans, flaxseed has the absolute most – at least 75 times more than any other plant food. This is important because lignans may have powerful antioxidant properties that can help block the damaging effects of free radicals. Lignans show particular promise for battling breast cancer. They do this by blocking the effects of oestrogen; exposure to oestrogen over time seems to increase breast cancer risk in some women. Even when oestrogen-sensitive tumours get a chance to grow, lignans exert a restraining influence that can slow or even halt their growth.

In a laboratory study, breast tumours in animals given flaxseed shrank by 50 per cent in seven weeks. In addition, it is rich in polyunsaturated fats, including omega–3 fatty acids. These appear to limit the body's production of prostaglandins, which, in large amounts, are thought to speed up tumour growths. And flaxseed is high in fibre, which quickly ushers harmful compounds out of the body.

Flaxseed oil comes in liquid and capsules, but you may want to skip the oil and just add flaxseed to your diet. The oil contains only trace amounts of the cancer-protective lignans because they are removed during processing. However, if you do decide to go with the supplement, stick with oil from the refrigerated section of your healthfood shop. Flaxseed oil degrades quickly when exposed to heat and light. Buy only oil that comes in an opaque bottle, and store it in the refrigerator as soon as you get home. Or, if you don't plan to use it right away, keep it in the freezer. Look for oils certified by a third party as organic. Also, many high-quality oils have a 'pressing date' listed on the bottles. If the oil was pressed more than six months ago, don't buy it.

Outwitting Osteoporosis

If you've ever pitied 'big-boned' women, save your sympathy. Their strength may protect them from osteoporosis, one of the most devastating age- and hormone-related processes women experience. It's a condition where the hormone-controlled process of bone breakdown speeds up as the bone-rebuilding process slows down. In the UK, 22.5 per cent of women of 50 and over have osteoporosis of the hip, and 50 per cent of women will suffer from osteoporosis by the age of 80. In Australia, half of all women over the age of 60 will suffer a fracture due to osteoporosis. In fact, the figures worldwide are fairly staggering. About 20 per cent of European women over 70 have had at least one wrist fracture. Some researchers predict that the number of hip fractures worldwide, now estimated at 1.8 million, could rise nearly fourfold by the year 2050 to more than six million, if present trends continue.

The more bone we build by the time we're in our twenties, the better prepared we are for bone loss that occurs with ageing and menopause. While our bones do begin to weaken as we age, osteoporosis is not inevitable. Doctors are sending the message to women that this is not

---

SUPER SUPPLEMENT CHECKLIST No. 5

By now, you know to take your calcium and vitamin D for strong, healthy bones. (And don't forget those weight-bearing exercises!) But there are plenty of other supplements that can help in the fight against osteoporosis and brittle bones. Here they are.

☐ Calcium   ☐ Nettle
☐ Vitamin D   ☐ Oat straw
☐ Magnesium   ☐ Dandelion leaf
☐ Vitamin K   ☐ Asian ginseng and ginger
☐ Horsetail   ☐ Alfalfa

---

really an illness of ageing, but rather an indication that the body isn't receiving enough calcium. Experts agree that that is never too late to strengthen your skeleton. Here are some supplements to help you avoid osteoporosis or, if you already have it, to slow its progress.

Calcium. Most women get about 500 milligrams or less of calcium a day from food. Much of that comes from dairy sources. If you happen to be lactose intolerant and therefore avoid most dairy products, you're probably getting even less than the average. In any case, you should probably have two or three times as much calcium as you're getting from food.

Almost every bit of calcium in your body is stored in your bones. There is also some in your blood, where it's used to regulate your heartbeat and keep muscle and nerve function and blood clotting at optimal levels. Your body's top priority is to maintain adequate levels of blood calcium. When these levels decline, your body will begin mining calcium from the next available source – your bones.

Knowing this, researchers have been probing to discover the optimal amount of calcium supplementation that most women need. At University Hospital in Ghent, Belgium, doctors found that a calcium intake of 1,500 milligrams a day helped protect postmenopausal women from bone loss. Another study, at Winthrop-University Hospital in New York, showed that giving 1,700 milligrams a day of calcium to women who were past menopause significantly slowed their rates of bone loss. Other studies show calcium's protective role against osteoporosis, but there are varying estimates of how much you need to take.

Dr Lorilee Schoenbeck, a naturopathic doctor, recommends 1,000 milligrams a day for women who are in menopause or have passed through it. Whatever amount you're taking, you want a supplement that provides the most easily absorbed form. Your body is better able to absorb and use calcium if it's in the form of citrate or aspartate. While some doctors say that you can get what you need from antacid tablets, Dr Schoenbeck notes that the calcium in antacids is less absorbable than calcium citrate. Another form you'll see on chemists' shelves is calcium carbonate, but that's the least absorbable, she says. (Taking this form with meals can increase absorption, however.)

Vitamin D. Vitamin D helps your body absorb supplemental calcium. A deficiency of D can lead to soft bones, which in turn can lead to fractures. Studies suggest that vitamin D is related to bone mineral density. Researchers at the Jean Mayer USDA Human Nutritional Research Center on Aging concluded that anywhere from 400 to 800 IU of vitamin D a day (taken with 1,000 to 1,500 milligrams of calcium) is necessary to minimize bone loss. For more information, see 'Vitamin D: the "Other" Bone-friendly Hormone' on page 92.

Magnesium. With regard to bone health, this mineral serves a different function from vitamin D. Magnesium is important because it transports calcium to the bones. It also helps convert vitamin D in the body to its active form.

A study in Israel found that 22 of 31 postmenopausal women who were given from 250 to 750 milligrams of magnesium for six months, then 250 milligrams a day for 18 months, increased their bone density by 1 to 8 per cent. Comparatively, a group of women who received no magnesium supplementation over the same period had rapid loss of bone density.

To work out how much magnesium you need, just take your calcium dosage and divide it in half. If you're taking 1,000 milligrams of calcium, for instance, you should take about 500 milligrams of magnesium. The least absorbable form of magnesium is magnesium oxide. You'll do better with magnesium aspartate.

Vitamin K. Vitamin K doesn't get much mention in the media, but it's very important for maintaining bone health. It helps reduce the amount of calcium you lose through urine. Vitamin K is also crucial to the formation of osteocalcin, a protein that is the matrix upon which calcium is put into the bone. 'Vitamin K is the foundation that calcium builds on,' says Dr Schoenbeck.

This vitamin is abundant in green leafy vegetables and whole grains. If your diet isn't rich in these foods, take a supplement that supplies the RNI of 1 microgram per kilo of body weight.

Horsetail. Horsetail is a reasonable source of silicon, one of the minerals that help give bones flexibility as well as strength, says Dr C. Leigh Broadhurst, a nutrition consultant and herbal researcher. To ensure that you get a pure, strong dose, she recommends using the liquid extract. Take two dropperfuls of extract in one mugful of water twice a day. Take it on an empty stomach, if possible, in the morning and in the evening.

Horsetail is also available in capsules, says Dr Allan Warshowsky, a gynaecologist. He recommends using capsules of standardized extract. Take 700 to 800 milligrams in capsule form twice a day.

Nettle. Nettle is an excellent source of magnesium and calcium, says Dr Warshowsky. Drink one dropperful of extract in a glass of water once or twice a day. Another way to take nettle is to buy standardized extract in capsule form. Take a 500-milligram capsule twice a day. People who have already developed signs of osteoporosis can double either dosage, he adds. Nettle tea is also available in healthfood shops.

Oat straw. Oat straw infusion is an excellent source of calcium and magnesium, according to herbalist Susun Weed. One particularly effective way to extract those minerals from the herb is to make a strong infusion, rather than a tea. Here are Susun's instructions. Put 30 g (1 oz) of dried oat straw in a large jar. Pour boiling water into the jar right to the top (approximately 1 l or 1¾ pints), put a tight lid on it, and let stand for at least four hours. Strain out the plant material and drink from 240 ml to 1 l (8 fl oz to 1¾ pints) a day as you like it, either hot or cold, she says. The taste is mild and mellow, but you can mix it with anything, even tea or coffee, if you wish. Refrigerate what you don't drink right away, but use it within 48 hours.

Dandelion leaf. Dandelion leaf has an abundance of minerals, including calcium, according to Dr Warshowsky. Take the extract according to the package directions twice a day. He recommends looking for a standardized extract.

Panax (Asian) ginseng and ginger. Like other root plants, ginseng and ginger can absorb plenty of minerals, especially boron, from the soil, says Dr Broadhurst. Ginseng has the added benefit of being an energy booster. Having energy can boost your enthusiasm for exercise, another important element of bone health. Take one 500-milligram capsule of each herb three times a day.

Alfalfa. The freshest way to ingest leafy green plants – your prime sources of bone-helping vitamin K – is to eat lots of salads, but an alfalfa supplement can help salad-phobic people get the green nutrients they need. Take four 500-milligram capsules of extract daily. Take two capsules in the morning and two at night, Dr Broadhurst suggests.

Another easy way to get more leafy greens in your diet, she adds, is to use the 'green drink' mixtures sold in healthfood shops, which combine everything from wheatgrass to various types of seaweed.

Congratulations! You've made it to the end of that long list of supplements. But we hope you noticed how many supplements fight several menopausal problems. And that means you don't have to take as many as it might seem at first. We suggest that you go back through this chapter, checklists in hand, and reread the sections that are most important to you. Note carefully how much, how often, and what form of each supplement to take for maximum effectiveness. Choose which supplements you want to try. (Of course, we hope *all* of you will take the basic vitamin/mineral supplement recommended on page 90, which gives you a great basis to begin adding specific supplements according to your needs.) Once you've made your list and checked it twice, it's time to move on to something that's every bit as important: managing your moods.

Chapter

5

MANAGING YOUR MOODS

To our mothers, the menopause marked the beginning of the end, the doorstep to old age. To us, it often represents the beginning of a whole new chapter in our lives, the opportunity to once again remake ourselves.

But into what?

'When it comes to facing menopause, the generations of women before us left no road maps,' says Stephanie DeGraff Bender, a clinical psychologist and author of *The Power of Perimenopause*.

They handled 'the Change' silently, privately, suffering through a bewildering range of symptoms, sometimes experiencing mood swings so unpredictable and severe that they feared for their sanity. At best, they might have taken some form of tranquillizer to get through unpredictable emotional swings.

Today we can do it differently. There are an assortment of modern-day, healthy ways to balance your moods and face the big 'M' with confidence and composure.

Working the Swing Shift

Your body temperature isn't the only thing that can suddenly switch from one extreme to the other during menopause. Some women feel very short-tempered and somewhat depressed. Even women who have experienced mood swings from premenstrual syndrome all their lives note that these are a bit more intense. 'They find it is much more noticeable than it used to be,' says Dr Lisa Domagalski, a gynaecologist.

Experts aren't sure what links mood changes to menopause. It could be an oestrogen connection, or it may have something to do with mood-altering brain chemicals, such as serotonin. Part of the difficulty may lie in sleep deprivation due to hot flushes and night sweats.

If your mood changes last a long time or impair your ability to work or function, or if you feel that you are slipping into a deep depression, see a doctor immediately. He will help you explore options such as medication and therapy. But if your mood changes are causing you (and those around you) only minor grief, try the following strategies to get your emotions back on an even keel.

Food and Your Mood

It's hardly news that many of us, when we're feeling down or irritated, seek emotional comfort in foods, particularly such 'comfort' foods as chocolate bars or cakes. But for some of us, comfort foods are anything but comforting. The very foods we eat to make ourselves feel better during mood swings may actually make us feel worse – listless, moody and fatigued.

Researchers have learned that what you eat can lift your mood or, if you make the wrong choices, sink it. Moreover, what you *don't* eat can have as great an impact as what you do. Here are two types of food that have the ability to keep you balanced.

Carbohydrates. In a study conducted by researchers at Harvard University and the Massachusetts Institute of Technology, women suffering from premenstrual mood swings were asked to drink about 225 ml (7½ fl oz) of a specially formulated high-carbohydrate drink once a month just before their periods. Within hours of having the drink, they experienced significant reductions in depression, anger and confusion, the researchers found.

While the women in the study consumed a specially made drink, you can get a similar amount of high carbohydrates by eating a small portion of a carbohydrate-rich food such as a pot of low-fat yoghurt, a baked potato or a handful of raisins or sultanas.

Omega-3 fatty acids. These substances, which are found in fish and certain other foods, are known mostly for keeping hearts healthy, but they may also help mood disorders. 'The brain is essentially made of fat,' explains Dr Joseph Hibbeln, a researcher at the National Institutes of Health. 'Some fats necessary for brain functioning – such as polyunsaturated fatty acids found in fish – cannot be manufactured by the body. You have to get them from diet.' So try to include more seafood in your diet. Dr Hibbeln also suggests using rapeseed oil while cooking as another way to increase your intake of omega-3s.

A 'NAVEL' IDEA

The next time you feel yourself floating off into a bad mood, stop for a second. Consider what is going on around you. Are you or someone close to you going through some kind of crisis, large or small? You might or might not be able to do anything to resolve it on the spot, but at least you'll know why you feel the way you do. Then, to help even out your mood, try this easy relaxation technique.

This is a simple exercise from qigong, an Eastern belief system in which the navel is the centre of existence. 'Qigong can refresh the body in a short period of time,' says Dr Leah J. Dickstein, director of attitudinal and behavioural medicine at the University of Louisville School of Medicine.

Sit with your palms cupped, the heels of your hands together at your navel. Open them very slowly. 'Think of pulling energy into your body,' says Dr Dickstein. 'Feel softness moving into the centre of your body, replacing bad feelings.' Repeat the entire process as often as you feel a need to.

Walk or Exercise Often

We told you to exercise in Chapter 4, The Menopause Exercise Plan. But just in case you somehow, ahem, skipped that chapter, we're going to give you a second chance. Because exercise – even gentle, steady exercise such as walking – really *can* work wonders on your mood. In a study conducted at Texas A&M University College of Medicine, women who walked for 20 minutes reported significant improvements in mood. 'Walking and exercise naturally increase the body's endorphins, chemicals in the body that make you feel good. That's where the "high" that people get from running comes from,' says Dr Domagalski.

But for exercise to work its magic, it has to be something you look forward to, not just another task on your already too long to-do list. Dr Sharon Brown, an assistant professor of physical education and exercise science, says she isn't particularly flexible, so yoga would frustrate her and be stressful. Running, however, is something she *does* do well, and it never fails to lift her spirits. 'Even better,' she says, 'is running with friends. This encourages me to exercise; plus, my friends help me find healthy perspectives and solutions to situations at work and with relationships.'

On the other side of the exercise equation is Dr Peggy Elam, a psychologist and yoga buff. She frequently recommends this ancient discipline to her clients as a way to deal with their own stress. The key is discovering what works best for you and finding the right balance.

Most important is doing something you like. If you're just starting out and aren't in very good shape, walking might be your best bet. If you're already fit and want to step up the pace a bit, you might consider a faster-paced aerobic work-out such as kickboxing.

For safe, gentle ways to lift your spirits through exercise, a blend of meditation and relaxation techniques, like yoga and t'ai chi, may be the answer. Almost anyone, at any age or any fitness level, can do them. (If you have a chronic condition, such as heart disease or back pain, or if you are pregnant, consult your doctor first. Once you get the go-ahead, let the instructor know your situation so that she can work with you.) For information on how to begin yoga or t'ai chi, see Chapter 9.

Take Time to Relax

In the early 1970s, Dr Herbert Benson at the Harvard Medical School devised the 'relaxation response'. This tension-releasing technique can help you through mood swings or periods of anxiety. Here's how to do it. Sit or lie down in a comfortable position and breathe deeply. Relax all your muscles. Think of a phrase or word that evokes feelings of relaxation for you, perhaps a word like *serene* or *calm*. Repeat the word in your mind every time you exhale. Practise this for 20 minutes once a day or 10 minutes twice a day, as well as any time you feel your mood beginning to change.

Master Mental Imagery

You can also use mental imagery to prevent shadows from darkening your days. Mental imagery is a quick and natural method to take control of the negative sensations that might arise during menopause. Dr Gerald Epstein, director of the American Institute for Mental Imagery and author of *Healing Visualizations*, offers this classic technique to relieve anxiety and irritability.

Sit in a comfortable chair, preferably with a high back and armrests for support. Place your arms on the armrests and your feet flat on the floor. Close your eyes and breathe out and then in three times slowly. Imagine yourself on a beach.

As you are looking at the sky far over the ocean, it begins to cloud over. You are hearing claps of thunder and seeing streaks of lightning as the storm gets closer and closer, gradually intensifying. Then, instead of letting loose, the dark clouds roll behind you, the sounds stop and the flashes cease. Looking out into the ocean, you see the sun come up in the sky and know that your symptoms have passed.

To stay in control of your emotions, do this imagery exercise three times a day at the same times each day. You can also practise it at the first sign of a symptom and continue until the difficulty is over.

If self-help techniques fail to control your mood swings – or if you experience mood swings on a daily basis – seek professional help. And

SOUND AWAY MENOPAUSAL MOODINESS

A mind-body technique called toning can help bring back harmony if you're experiencing menopausal mood swings and other symptoms.

'The use of the voice is a built-in tool that releases emotional tension from your body,' says Don Campbell, a sound researcher and director of the Mozart Effect Resource Center. 'A daily practice of toning, which is making a sound with an elongated vowel for an extended period, can improve your overall state of mind.'

Toning is a great help for releasing and harmonizing your emotions during and following menopause because it moves your emotions through your body so that you don't feel pent-up, vulnerable or ready to explode, he explains. When your body responds to the vibration you are creating, your hormone levels even out.

Don tells of a student who claims that she benefited so greatly from a toning practice that she could stop hormone replacement therapy and say goodbye to her hot flushes.

Here is a brief outline of Don Campbell's Five-Day Toning Class. Do each exercise for about five minutes, holding the tone continually with natural breaths in between. If you enjoy the experience, repeat it whenever you need some relaxation or reviving.

Day 1 – hum: sit comfortably, close your eyes, and hum – not a melody, but

don't be embarrassed to ask for medical or psychiatric advice; you might have an underlying condition whose treatment eliminates mood swings.

The Power of Positive Thinking

It's not a compliment to be called a Pollyanna. The little orphan girl who brimmed with boundless cheer has come to epitomize the cockeyed optimist who doesn't quite see reality for what it is. The fact is, positive thinking has had a bad press. We tend to trivialize positive emotions such as hope, joy and contentment.

'People think they're wasting their time when they're experiencing positive emotions,' explains Dr Barbara Fredrickson, a psychologist. 'The possible benefits of positive emotions seem undervalued in cultures like

a pitch that feels comfortable. Relax your jaw and feel the energy of the hum warming up and energizing your entire body.

Day 2 – ah sound: the *ah* sound immediately evokes a relaxation response. Whenever you feel a great deal of stress and tension, relax your jaw and make a quiet *ah*. In your office or other places where toning may disturb others, you can simply close your eyes, breathe out and think the *ah*.

Day 3 – ee sound: the *ee* sound can awaken your mind and body, functioning as a kind of sonic caffeine. When you feel drowsy while driving or are sluggish in the afternoon, making a high *ee* sound will stimulate your brain and keep you alert. The *ee* tone is also good for releasing tension. Just don't practise it if you have a headache as the increased activity in your brain may make it worse.

Day 4 – oh sound: the *oh* tone is a great tool for an instant tune-up. Your body responds to the *oh* by normalizing your skin temperature, breathing and heart rate as well as releasing muscle tension and increasing brain waves.

Day 5 – experimental singing: start at the lowest part of your voice and let it glide upward, like a very slow elevator. Make vowel sounds that are relaxing and that arise effortlessly from your jaw or throat. Allow your voice to resonate throughout your body. Now explore the ways in which you can 'massage' parts of your skull, throat and chest with long vowel sounds.

ours, which cast hard work and self-discipline as virtues, and leisure and pleasures as sinful.'

But research shows that feeling good *is* good. And if we want to find our way to natural calm and balanced emotions, we need to nurture what is best in ourselves.

Positive psychology shifts the focus from what's *wrong* with us to what's *right* with us. The latest research in this fledgling field has shown that cultivating optimism, joy, contentment, interest and other positive feelings and attitudes can help prevent and treat problems that can cause mood swings, such as anxiety, depression and stress–related health problems. For tips on how to turn your thinking around, see 'Adopt a "Glass Half Full" Attitude' on page 138.

ADOPT A 'GLASS HALF FULL' ATTITUDE

So how do we learn to become a 'glass half full' type of person instead of a 'glass half empty' person? First, understand what that means.

'Positive emotions are more than the absence of negative emotions,' says Dr Barbara Fredrickson, a psychologist.

One of the misunderstandings about this way of thinking is that all you have to do is put on a happy face, says psychologist Dr Dacher Keltner. But thinking positively involves taking an alternative approach, and that requires a great deal of hard work. It's difficult and taxing, he says, but ultimately rewarding.

These six simple steps will start your transformation.

Put on your rose-tinted glasses. Studies show that people in difficult situations who are able to reframe their circumstances in a more positive light cope with stress better.

For instance, AIDS care-givers who focused on the value of their efforts and commented on how their care-giving activities demonstrated their love and preserved the dignity of their ill partners fared best, says Dr Susan Folkman, professor of medicine and co-director of the Center for AIDS Prevention Studies at the University of California.

To get a rosier view of your own life, look at the lessons you've learned from a bad situation, suggests Dr Folkman. Or simply give yourself a well-deserved pat on the back when you've just endured a very stressful situation. Say to yourself, 'I didn't realize I could do that.'

Act happy. We can *act* ourselves into a more positive frame of mind, says Dr David G. Myers, author of *The Pursuit of Happiness*. Research has shown that simply manipulating your face into a smiling expression by holding a pen in your teeth can make you feel better. On the other hand, hold the pen in your lips, and you activate the frowning muscles. 'Scowl and the whole world seems to scowl back,' he says.

'Going through the motions can trigger the emotions,' says Dr Myers. 'So . . . put on a happy face. Talk as if you feel positive, optimistic and outgoing,' even if you don't.

Take control of your time. Happy people feel in control of their lives. But stress makes you feel as if your life is out of control. 'We often overestimate how much we will accomplish in any given day, which leaves us feeling frustrated,' says Dr Myers.

When you start feeling like this, it's best to focus on immediate goals. Make a to-do list for the day. But make sure the tasks are specific and small, such as

'Post letter to Aunt Hilda', not 'Organize my cupboard'. The more, the better. And then (and this is key) take *pleasure* in crossing each one off as you accomplish it. 'It reduces anxiety and helps you regain a sense of control because you feel more effective. And that's no small thing,' says Dr Folkman.

Laugh it up. 'Laughter is a good thing in times of stress. That's why people often laugh at unlikely times – at a funeral, for example,' explains Dr Keltner. He interviewed mourners and noted how often they laughed and expressed positive emotions. Two years later, he interviewed them again and found that those who had displayed the most positive emotions were the least likely to have experienced depression and anxiety. In times of stress, laughter reduces the physiological reaction to stress and feelings of anxiety and helps people form stronger bonds with others.

Be social. We feel better when we're interacting with others, says Dr Myers. So give priority to close relationships. If you're married, resolve to nurture your relationship, to not take your partner for granted. Treat your husband with the same kindness that you display to others. To rejuvenate your affections, behave lovingly, play together and share common interests.

Savour positive moments. We might not realize it, but even when we're under stress, we also experience positive moments. In 1,794 interviews with AIDS care-givers, Dr Folkman was surprised to find that 99.5 per cent were able to recall a positive event – something that had made them feel good and helped them get through the day.

So tune in to those moments when they happen. 'They give you a moment of relief – like relaxing a muscle that's been tense for a long time. That brief moment can be restorative,' says Dr Folkman. It could be receiving a compliment, observing a beautiful sunset, or hearing your teenager say, 'Thanks, Mum'. Or it could be something planned, such as a special meal or a get-together with friends.

Delight in those ordinary but positive moments in your day, and amplify them, says Dr Folkman. For instance, pause when you see that sunset, and pay attention to this bright spot in your day. Or take time for a period of reflection at the end of the day and think about all the moments that day that made you feel good. This reinforces what's meaningful and valuable in your life, motivating you and building self-confidence. In short, paying attention to positive emotions helps breed more positive emotion.

'Instead of focusing on what you might perceive as negative about menopause, you can say, "Now is the time to take better care of myself, eat more healthily, get enough sleep and get rid of what is toxic in my life",' she advises.

Have the Last Laugh

Dwindling fertility hormones may be an unstoppable fact of life, but you can certainly boost your 'feel good' hormones. Research shows that laughing produces beneficial physiological effects because it reduces the release of stress hormones from the adrenal gland while increasing the production of endorphins, the body's natural feel-good hormones.

'Humour can reduce anxiety, soften anger, lighten depression and raise your tolerance for pain. In all seriousness, laughter is beneficial for your body, mind and soul, particularly when you are going through difficult times,' says Dr David Simon, medical director of the Chopra Center for Well Being, and author of *Vital Energy*. (For tips on how to entertain your playful spirit, see 'What's So Funny?' on the opposite page.)

Oestrogen and Depression

'Oestrogen makes women feel good,' says Dr Martha Louise Elks, a professor of medicine. It seems to raise levels of the feel-good hormone serotonin, making us mellower and more flexible in how we react to whatever life throws us. 'We still notice life's injustices, but we're not so bothered by them,' Dr Elks says. 'We say, "Yeah, he's a pig – men are pigs. So what?"'

Try that philosophy during a menopausal state, when your oestrogen levels are low or erratic. Then your response is likely to be 'Yeah, he's a pig' as we slam the door/throw the plate/storm out of the room. Studies have shown that depression and even suicide attempts are more frequent during oestrogen lulls.

Conventional treatments for depression include a variety of antidepressant drugs, psychotherapy or a combination of both. Oestrogen replacement therapy also seemed to help women with perimenopausal and postmenopausal depression, according to a study, published in the *Journal of the American Menopause Society*, that was a review of the medical literature on women and depression.

While you should seek help from a qualified mental health expert for

WHAT'S SO FUNNY?

Here are some ideas for entertaining your playful spirit.

- Create your own compilation videos of film clips and television episodes that make you laugh. That way, you'll have them on hand when you need to lighten up. You can also hire or buy compilation tapes such as *Friends* reruns or Monty Python sketches and watch bits of them every night.
- Stock up on silliness. Find joke books and comics that are laugh-out-loud funny, and keep them by your bed, in the bathroom, on the refrigerator – anywhere that you can always see them.
- Take a stand-up artist for a ride. Get cassettes or compact discs of comedians that you can listen to in your car so that long drives actually cheer you up.
- Sign up for a free joke-a-day service on the internet via e-mail. Just type 'joke' into your web browser, or try logging on to websites such as *www.laugh-of-the-day.com*, *www.funs.co.uk* or *www.laughs.com.au*.
- Catch the bug. Laughter is not only the best medicine; it's contagious, too! When you read a humorous anecdote, quote or cartoon, post it on your notice board or another place where you'll be able to share others' enjoyment.
- See the comical side of the change. Read a funny book about menopause, such as *The Noisy Passage* by Marie Evans and Ann Shakeshaft.
- Instead of the typical dinner and a film, why not take a friend or your partner to comedy clubs or social clubs that feature a comedian for the night's entertainment?
- When you host or attend parties, suggest funny-bone-tickling interactive games like Pictionary, Cranium, Taboo and Balderdash.

any sign of depression, there may be some things you can do to help lift the clouds of mild to moderate depression.

Move for your mood. Just as physical activity helps to balance mood swings, it can also prevent and treat depression. Researchers don't know exactly why exercise helps, but they suggest it may enhance our sense of mastery so we feel more mentally and physically in control. Aerobic activity may also help vent pent-up frustration. And mood-enhancing endorphins (runner's high) released during exercise could also be involved. Aim for at least 30 minutes of exercise most days. If you want, you can break it into three sets of 10 minutes each.

Expand your exercise horizons. Yoga is an excellent depression remedy. For one thing, if you take a class, you'll bond with others, says Dr

ST JOHN'S WORT TO THE RESCUE

If you've tried Prozac or some other prescription antidepressant, but don't like the side-effects (lower sexual desire being one), you might want to consider St John's wort.

St John's wort has received a lot of publicity as 'natural Prozac' over the years. Studies have found that St John's wort alleviates mild to moderate depression as effectively as prescription antidepressants. Scientists aren't sure how St John's wort works but speculate that it increases levels of the mood-elevating chemical serotonin.

One ingredient, hypericin, is believed to be responsible for the herb's anti-depressant effects, but newer research indicates that St John's wort might contain many other active ingredients.

'It's not just one molecule with one effect, as with synthetic drugs,' says Dr Harold Bloomfield, author of *Hypericum and Depression*. 'St John's wort has many active ingredients, and they all work together.'

Widely used to relieve depression, St John's wort has some definite advantages over synthetic drugs. It isn't addictive, causes no withdrawal symptoms, and can be safely mixed with alcohol. Nor does it produce the side-effects commonly associated with antidepressant drugs, such as nausea, gastrointestinal distress and lowered sex drive. 'Prescription antide-pressants aren't necessary to treat mild depression,' says Dr Bloomfield.

Ellen Kamhi, author of *Cycles of Life: Herbs and Energy Techniques for Women*. Also, some movements and breathing exercises in yoga can stimulate glands to release mood-enhancing hormones. (For more on yoga, see page 285.)

Illuminate yourself. 'Before we use any herbs or supplements, we need to find out what's causing the depression,' says Dr Kamhi. Sometimes it's something relatively simple, such as lack of sunlight, which can be treated with a light box. These devices shine full-spectrum light on your face, simulating natural sunlight. Light treatment should be considered even before the use of herbs, she says, because there are no chemicals or toxicities in light, and you can operate a light box at work or at home. Use this treatment only in consultation with your doctor, who can explain proper use of the box and set up an appropriate treatment schedule for you.

'St John's wort is the first thing I prescribe for depression,' says Dr Hyla Cass, assistant clinical professor of psychiatry at the UCLA School of Medicine. 'It may not help every woman, but it's unlikely ever to hurt anyone.'

If your doctor has ruled out serious depression, you may want to give St John's wort a try. However, check with your doctor first if you are taking any other medications because it may affect the way they work. Here's what you need to know.

Take just what you need, and no more. Doctors who prescribe St John's wort usually suggest 300 milligrams three times a day. Look for products with 0.3 per cent extract of hypericin.

The best dose, says Dr Cass, 'is the lowest one that produces results'. She suggests starting with the recommended dosage, then tapering after a few months to find the optimal dosage. Some people will find they can eventually stop taking the herb completely without a recurrence of symptoms.

Take it with food. Some women experience nausea the first few days, which usually vanishes when the herb is taken with food.

Wear sunscreen, wraparound sunglasses and a hat if you go outdoors. Evidence suggests that St John's wort may increase sensitivity to the sun if you're light-skinned.

Don't expect instant results. 'Like prescription antidepressants, St John's wort often takes three or four weeks before it kicks in,' says Dr Bloomfield.

Brew a soothing tea. 'My favourite antidepressant is a tea made of Siberian ginseng and rosebuds – it immediately lifts your spirits,' says Dr Kamhi. Get Siberian ginseng from a healthfood shop in the form of the whole root, in a tea bag or in a capsule.

Welcome support. Nourish emotional and physical improvements among other women experiencing menopause. Much research has shown that a support group can be an essential element in enhancing both mental and physical health. In a ten-year American study at Stanford University study of women with advanced stages of breast cancer, researchers found that the women who were in a support group lived twice as long as those who were not in a support group.

'The group process offers wonderful energy to support change,' says counsellor Louise Hay, an expert in creative power and personal growth and author of 27 bestsellers, including *You Can Heal Your Life*. A menopause support group can be a focused opportunity for women to share their experiences on the sometimes unpredictable path of menopause. But don't use your group to sit around and say 'isn't it awful…' Share ideas of ways to cope. Use the group as a stepping-stone in your growth process.

Making New Connections

Social support can step in and buffer us against the abrasive effects of gloomy feelings, depression and mood swings.

And when it comes to making those stress-reducing connections, women have the edge. We give one another more frequent and effective social support, we're quicker to provide help when a friend is depressed or sad, and we're more satisfied overall than men with our personal connections.

In fact, new studies suggest we have our own, unique way to deal with stress, called 'tend and befriend', and it's more effective than the fight-or-flight mechanism we'd previously been thought to use.

Reducing Stress with Friendship

'Social support is emotionally nurturing, and if it's emotionally nurturing, it's going to be physically nurturing – in other words, the classic

ALLEVIATE ANXIETY WITH ACUPRESSURE

A few minutes of acupressure, the fine art of finger pressure, can help ease your body and mind.

If you are experiencing feelings of anxiety as you approach mid-life, or if you find yourself generally feeling stressed-out, acupressure can provide you with calming relief, says David Nickel, a doctor of oriental medicine and a licensed acupuncturist.

How does it work? A practitioner could give you a lengthy explanation about how acupressure restores complex energetic pathways in your body. But in Western terms, pressing your fingers or knuckles in the right places improves circulation throughout your body, including your brain. The resulting flood of minerals, enzymes, oxygen and pleasure chemicals brings relief from muscular and emotional tension.

A quick way to relieve minor anxiety is to apply pressure to the Spirit Gate point, located on the outside of your wrist, below the first crease and in line with your little finger. Press on this spot until you get an aching sensation similar to when you hit your funny bone.

Maintain this pressure for 15 to 30 seconds, then release. For optimal results, do not work the same spot more than two or three times a day.

For help in getting started, see page 270.

mind–body connection,' says psychologist Dr Patricia McWhorter. More specifically, social support has many benefits.

Here are a few of the best.

It calms. Stress produces physiological responses, including increased heart rate, breathing and blood pressure, that over time can harm emotional and physical health. 'And social support cuts off this dysfunctional cycle,' says Dr Judith C. Tingley, a psychologist.

One study found that women experienced high blood pressure and increased heart rates only when they performed stressful tasks alone, compared with those who worked with or were in the presence of a female friend or even a female stranger. In the latter cases, heart rate and blood pressure responses were minimal. Just having another woman in the room, whether she was a stranger or a friend, reduced stress.

This calming power appears to work over the long term, too. People who have social connections bounce back more quickly from surgery and illnesses than those without support.

It takes a load off. When you have solid social connections, you have people who are prepared to help, whether it's a lift to work or someone to care for your children in an emergency. 'There are people there to say, "Don't worry, we've got this covered", which reduces stress,' says Dr David Posen, a public speaker and author of *Always Change a Losing Game*.

Social support might also help stop stress from starting in the first place. For example, if you face work conflict but have sufficient social support from your colleagues, you'll be less likely to view the problem as stressful.

It dissolves distress. We feel much better when we talk things through. 'And when we hear ourselves talk, we can often get to the root of what's bothering us without the listener saying a word,' says Dr Posen.

It validates. If someone listens empathetically and says things like 'Oh, that must be hard' or 'I agree' or 'That happened to me, too', it makes us feel better, says Mark Gorkin, a social worker and author of *Practice Safe Stress*. 'You begin to feel like you're not alone or a freak of nature after all,' he says.

It boosts self-esteem. 'Anything that threatens our self-esteem (for instance, someone threatening or criticizing us) produces a stress response,' says Dr Posen. Our social connections help us feel better about ourselves – good friends make us feel good, and we feel as if we're part of a larger whole. 'And as self-esteem improves, stress diminishes,' he says.

It lingers. 'Social support instills a kind of inner foundation – you carry around the beliefs and sharing that you receive from your social connections even when they're not there, like that great teacher you had at school who remains a role model throughout your life,' says Mark Gorkin.

Female Friends: the Ultimate Connection

Research shows that social support from women, rather than from men, is more stress relieving to both sexes.

A study at the University of California recorded the blood pressure responses of men and women who gave a five-minute impromptu speech to either a male or a female audience. Even though the audiences behaved identically, the speakers had lower blood pressure when they talked before a female audience. 'We're not sure why this is,' says study researcher Dr Nicholas Christenfeld, an associate professor of psychology. 'But we suspect it may be because the speakers interpreted the support differently when it came from women. When it came from men, the support was interpreted as "I understand what you're saying, and you're making good points", but when it came from a woman, it was interpreted as "I like you as a person".'

It seems that females are just more socially wired than males are. 'Our connections are more naturally feelings-based,' says Dr McWhorter. A landmark anthropology study illustrated this difference, she says. Researchers watched two opposing tribes of chimpanzees. The males from each tribe waited at the imaginary line of territory, throwing rocks and chasing one another away. Meanwhile, the females sneaked into one another's trees, where they secretly bonded, groomed one another and played with one another's infants.

Finding Your Own Connections

Although simply being a woman provides an advantage when it comes to making connections, there's more you can do. Here are some ways to build social networks (or strengthen the ones you already have).

Be supportive yourself. Our mothers told us when we were little: 'To have a friend, you have to be a friend'. The amount of social support we give is as important as how much we get. Follow these guidelines to be a good supporter.

- Ask questions, and show interest in what the other person has to say.
- Just listen. 'Don't judge or tell the person what she should do – that's the last thing we need when we need social support,' says Dr McWhorter.
- Nurture your friendships with regular phone calls, invitations and support.
- When something is shared with you in confidence, don't tell your five best friends.

Focus on quality, not quantity. A study at Yale University found that people with just a few friends who felt loved and supported had fewer coronary blockages than those with many friends who felt less loved and supported. Here are five characteristics necessary for high-quality social connections.

Compassion. 'To feel supported, you have to feel cared for and understood,' says Dr Tingley.

Unconditional love. 'You need to feel safe to be vulnerable, silly and free to let it all hang out,' says Dr McWhorter.

Accessibility. Solid social support is there for you whenever you need it, even at four o'clock on a Monday morning.

Trustworthiness. 'You want someone who won't ridicule you or let the whole world know about your problem,' says Dr Linda Sapadin, a psychologist.

Honesty. Someone who constantly tells you you're wonderful isn't going to be much help. 'Find someone who can listen but also be objective,' says Mark Gorkin.

Know what to avoid. When it comes to confiding in someone, it's smart to look out for the red flags. Dr Posen recommends you keep it to yourself when you notice any of these five traits.

Cattiness. Someone who reveals others' confidences to you is also likely to reveal yours to them.

Lack of empathy. If you're having relationship problems because of your infertility, a happily married woman with three children may not be able to empathize. Choose someone you can relate to on this particular issue.

Self-centredness. The woman who immediately switches the focus of the conversation from your problem to herself probably won't be much help.

Disinterest. If she seems impatient when you're talking, she probably isn't interested.

Insensitivity. If she's uncaring when she talks about others, she's probably not going to be too caring with you either.

Start with what you have. 'You might not have to build a support system – you might just have to start being more open with the people

AGE GRACEFULLY

Is your attitude about growing older a fair one, or is it ruled by society's stereotypes?

'It's no wonder so many menopausal women get depressed, living in the context of an "ageist" culture, which assumes that growing older is an inevitable decline into incapacity, fatigue and despondency,' says Dr Alice D. Domar, Director of the women's health programmes for the division of behavioural medicine at Harvard Medical School.

Certain changes do tend to occur at mid-life. For example, losing weight becomes harder, libido fluctuates and social and family roles may shift. But none of this should mean menopausal women can't feel attractive, be fully sexual, come into their creativity, develop careers or redefine relations with loved ones in ways that are profoundly gratifying, says Dr Domar.

Your distorted ideas about ageing might come from someone else's fear or stereotype. 'In other words, if your mind is a bus, who is driving it? Is it your boss? Your mother-in-law? Your father? A partner you split up from years ago? The media? For people who have negative beliefs running around their heads,' says Dr Domar, 'the usual answer to "who is driving your bus" is anyone but themselves.'

Have the courage to question the origins of your negative impressions about menopausal and postmenopausal years. Then you can take the wheel and follow your self-guided directions on the road of maturity that leads to peace of mind and vitality.

you already know,' says Dr Posen. Your 'fun friend' (with whom you've never pondered anything deeper than what kind of martini to order) could turn out to be a great listener.

Talk to strangers. 'It's often easier to confide in strangers than friends because you don't have to worry about them telling others you know, and you don't have to worry about damaging their opinion of you,' says Dr Sapadin. Support groups and group therapy provide excellent opportunities for stranger interaction.

Join a group. If you run for exercise, join a running group. If you read, join a book club. If you want to do something for the community, volunteer. 'You'll meet people with common interests, and they'll also be doing some things you're not doing, which can challenge you to stretch and grow,' says Mark Gorkin.

Go online. The internet helps build social bridges among diverse groups of people. 'In some chat groups, people come together and are honest with one another,' says Mark. 'They gradually open up and meet people with whom they can create a one-on-one relationship.'

A study reported in the *American Journal of Community Psychology* gave 42 single women computer-mediated social support (CMSS) concerning parenting issues. The online discussions revealed close personal relationships among the women, and the mothers who regularly participated in CMSS experienced less parenting stress.

Online groups are also great if you want to remain anonymous. But as with all web information, consider the source and be cautious. Visit the site a few times before you decide to join.

With all these mood-enhancing options to choose from, we hope you're starting to feel better already. And once you start feeling better, you might find yourself starting to think about all sorts of pleasurable things again . . . such as sex. To find out how to have the best time of your life in bed (or any other place you find appealing), turn to Chapter 6.

Chapter

6

MAKING SEX GREAT AGAIN

IF YOUR SEX LIFE HAS BECOME COMPROMISED BY MID–LIFE CRISES, painful intercourse, chronic disease, a change in your marital status, or any of the hormonal changes of menopause, don't bottle up your desires. Denying your passionate nature is a sure way to sap one of the most sublime pleasures from your life – not to mention your partner's. Besides, frequent sex in mid–life and beyond is actually quite good for you and can even help manage some symptoms of the menopause.

According to the results of a University of Chicago study, women who engage in sex once a week have higher oestrogen levels. In fact, women with sporadic, rather than weekly, sexual activity had a 50 per cent chance of developing severely low oestrogen levels. The benefit of consistent indulging might very well translate to fewer hot flushes, less vaginal dryness, better odds of withstanding osteoporosis and slower ageing, says Patricia Love, a marriage and family therapist and relationship consultant and co-author of *Hot Monogamy*.

The specific reasons that sex is good for keeping ageing women youthful are a bit complex, says Dr Love. It all begins with oxytocin, the chemical that triggers orgasm (also released during breastfeeding) and causes you to bond with your partner, she explains. Bonding encourages more touching, and that in turn releases endorphins, the body's natural 'opiates'. When this happens often, Dr Love says that it colours your life with a sense of tranquillity and happiness that ultimately offsets ageing, both emotionally and physically.

Dr Love suggests maintaining weekly sexual relations even if you don't always feel like it. 'You might just think of sex as meeting your partner's needs. What you don't realize is that it's also good for you because it sends a signal to your body that says, "I'm still young, alive and vibrant".'

Another dividend is that regular sexual activity stimulates the vaginal lining to produce natural lubricants, keeping vaginal dryness at bay. And if your own lubrication is inadequate, sex encourages you to apply creams and moisturizers, which further maintain vaginal health. To reap that benefit, you don't necessarily need a partner. Masturbating twice a week can produce the same results.

But all of this begs the question: if sex at mid-life is so good for us, why aren't we having orgasms every day? Surveys show that almost one in three women over 50 hasn't had sex in the past year. The same is true for about one in seven over 40.

If this statistic applies to you, then let this chapter help you open the door to a more vibrant – and fulfilling – sex life.

Make the Most of a Mid-life Crisis

For many women, menopause signals the beginning of a whole new stage in life. Mid-life affords us time to begin thinking about autonomy and individuality, about expressing who we really are. 'I see women becoming more assertive, in a positive way, and more active. We move beyond our traditional roles as nurturers and begin putting ourselves first,' says Dr Carol Landau, a clinical professor of psychiatry and human behaviour and co-author of *The Complete Book of Menopause*. That could mean speaking up more at home and at work, pursuing a more meaningful career or doing voluntary work, choosing new hobbies or making new friends – or taking other steps that bring new meaning to your daily life.

At the same time, a woman might also look more critically at the

PUT A SLANT ON GREAT SEX

As women age, their uterine muscles tend to weaken and sag downwards, undermining full sensations of intercourse or even causing the embarrassment of leaking urine in the heat of the moment. But you can battle gravity by keeping the supporting muscles in the pubic region toned with daily pelvic floor (Kegels) exercises, says Dr Helen Healy, a naturopathic doctor. For the best results, do them while lying on a slantboard, a padded piece of exercise equipment that allows you to lie down on an adjustable incline.

Kegel exercises consist of contracting and relaxing the pubococcygeal muscle, which is used to stop and start the flow of urine. When this muscle is in good working order, the tissues surrounding it remain healthier and better oxygenated, says Dr Healy. By strengthening it, menopausal women can maintain better control and even better vaginal lubrication. Better yet, women report improved sex lives and more intense orgasms after doing Kegels routinely.

Dr Healy suggests lying on a slantboard set at a 25- to 30-degree angle (with one end raised about 60 cm/2 ft) with your head at the low end. While in that position, squeeze the pubococcygeal muscle hard and hold it for about five seconds, then release and relax for three seconds. Always do this on an empty stomach to prevent a potential hiatus hernia. For optimal benefits, work up to 100 squeezes per day. (Not all of them need to be done on a slantboard!) The beauty of Kegels is that you can pretty much do them anywhere – even sitting at the dinner table or in front of the TV, and no one will know.

---

quality of intimacy in her relationships with her partner, her children and her friends, and feel a need for a deeper connection. This type of inward assessment can bring on a wave of growing pains that can strain not only a good sex life but the marriage itself.

And in truth not all marriages survive mid-life changes. The divorce rate among middle-aged people is second only to the rate among younger couples who've been married seven years or less. If one partner has felt alienated for years and has stayed only to raise the kids or out of economic necessity, then mid-life can present an opportunity to leave a bad situation and start again.

But do feelings of discontentment necessarily mean that you've made all the wrong choices, or that to be happy you need to get divorced, lose weight or take a handsome lover? Of course not! Instead, a strong sense of restlessness is a loud signal that it's time to pay attention to your inner needs, not necessarily a sign that your life needs a complete overhaul. Small or gradual changes may make all the difference.

Mid-life Crises: What You Can Do for Yourself

To help you sort out your unhappiness and decide what to do, experts offer this advice.

Let the big questions simmer. Set aside some time to ask yourself questions about your life, and then let the answers rise to the surface. 'I ask myself if I'm doing what I really want to be doing. If I'm still happy with my marriage, my job, my social life,' says Dr Janice Levine, a clinical psychologist. 'The questions just simmer in the back of my mind. I notice that little red flags go up if I find I'm doing things that I really don't want to be doing.'

In the same way, little green flags may go up when you are doing what pleases you most. If you pay attention to the red and green flags, you could have an 'aha' moment, when you recognize choices that are working for or against you.

Select a confidante. For most women, the single most important help at mid-life is having a close friend in whom you can confide. Choose someone who can listen without having her own agenda. For instance, if you are married and need to talk over doubts about your relationship, do not confide in a woman who is in the midst of a separation herself.

Put regret in its place. At mid-life, many women feel at least some regrets. Some point you towards important actions, such as making peace with your parents or siblings. But others can take on a life of their own, with no resolution. If you find yourself ruminating about the road not taken, it might be time to forgive yourself for simply being human. (After all, if you decided to raise three children and work part-time instead of becoming a research chemist or a concert pianist, remind yourself that you made a great choice. No one can do everything. Put superwoman to rest.)

KEEP UP WITH CONTRACEPTION

When it comes to birth control, better safe than sorry is a rule not to break when you're approaching menopause.

Sex without risk of pregnancy could make those annoying menopausal symptoms seem worthwhile. But don't throw your contraceptives away after your first hot flush. 'Pregnancy is possible during the perimenopausal years,' warns Dr Brian Walsh, assistant professor of obstetrics and gynaecology and reproductive biology at Harvard Medical School. 'Admittedly, the risk is low, but it's not zero.'

An unplanned pregnancy on the brink of menopause could prove both physically and emotionally burdensome, so it's essential to use birth control every time you have intercourse. Some women assume that the rhythm method is a good option during perimenopause, especially since irregular ovulation lowers their chances of conceiving; however, the accompanying irregular menstrual cycles also make it difficult to judge 'safe' times, so the rhythm method is still unreliable.

Barrier methods, which include diaphragms and condoms, are wise choices, says Dr Walsh. Spermicidal formulas, however, can irritate sensitive vaginal tissue and should be avoided if vaginal dryness, typical of menopause, is a problem. Women who can safely take oestrogen may benefit from low-dose birth control pills, which also offer symptomatic relief from hot flushes and menstrual irregularities.

When do contraceptives become extraneous? After your periods have stopped completely for a year, says Dr Walsh. But since on-again-off-again cycles can make the determination difficult, it's best to consult your doctor before you stop taking the Pill.

Restoring Intimacy

Trying to hide mid-life questioning from your partner won't work – and could be dangerous for your marriage, experts caution. 'He will probably see changes in your behaviour before you do,' says Dr Levine. You might start acting distant, lose interest in activities you've shared for years, stop seeing old friends as often, even change your wardrobe or your hairstyle. He's bound to notice and wonder what's up. And, if you are avoiding sex, that could very well be misinterpreted as rejection by your lover.

More important, resisting change out of fear that your marriage will be altered short-changes both you and your relationship. 'If you hold back in an effort to keep everything the same, your need for change might express itself in unhealthy ways. You might grow to resent your husband, become depressed, even spend money recklessly or have an affair,' notes Dr Levine.

So speak up. For all you know, he might be experiencing similar feelings. 'A lot of couples go through mid-life changes at the same time,' Dr Landau explains. How men and women deal with change is different, though. While a man might distract himself, a woman might be more likely to want to talk things out.

Think through your frustrations before starting a conversation. If you feel bored with your sex life or your marriage, don't simply blame your husband. Ask yourself why. Perhaps you always imagined that married life would bring a certain kind of excitement, but that hasn't materialized. And so it may be time to give up an unrealistic expectation. Or perhaps the two of you are stuck in old routines – maybe you've made love the same way for decades, or done the same things every weekend for years. It might be time to try something new.

Once you've thought through what you really want to say, try talking to your partner in a non-threatening way about your hopes and frustrations. Pick a time when the two of you are relaxed, not tired or rushed. It's usually best to talk about sex outside the bedroom. And be specific about what you want from him, and ready to suggest some alternative activities.

Once you have opened up the lines of communication, together you can experiment with solutions. Perhaps, for example, he needs to understand that at mid-life a woman requires a longer period of foreplay, and you can learn seductive massage techniques together. Maybe he'll finally take you on that romance-revving holiday or lingerie shopping date that he's been procrastinating about for the 30 years of your marriage.

The fact is, for many women, menopause becomes a liberating time to experiment with different sexual behaviours, such as oral sex. Communicate – and you're on the road to joining the ranks of women who report their postmenopausal years as their best sex years.

Overcome Menopausal Symptoms

Many women try to keep certain menopausal symptoms private as long as possible, but that can be difficult to do in the bedroom, where many of the most physically intimate moments of the day occur. Here, then, is the best advice for dealing with the two symptoms most likely to interfere with your sex life: hot flushes and vaginal dryness.

Steamy Sex without Hot Flushes

You want hot sex, but instead you have hot flushes. Don't despair. You have enough stress to manage during menopause without straining your most intimate, supporting relationship. If hot flushes and night sweats leave you less than lustful, consider the following solutions.

Take a herbal chiller. Medical research suggests that black cohosh, a popular herbal remedy, contains oestrogen-like substances that help relieve menopausal symptoms, especially hot flushes. Anecdotal reports suggest that black cohosh also can increase menopausal women's sex drives, says Dr Kimberly Windstar, a naturopathic doctor.

But unlike conventional hormone therapy, black cohosh doesn't raise blood levels of oestrogen. This makes the herb a boon particularly for women who have experienced breast cancer because black cohosh quells hot flushes without increasing the risk of recurrence.

Experts recommend a daily dose of 40 milligrams, taken for no more than 6 months. Some women find that one 40-milligram capsule is enough, says Dr Windstar, while others might need to discuss increasing their dosages with their practitioners for best results. Because black cohosh is such a potent herb, it's best to consult your doctor before taking it, especially if you've had breast cancer.

Make love between flushes. Hot flushes seem to be most frequent from 6 am to 8 am and from 6 pm to 10 pm, explains Dr Landau. So if hot flushes are a big impediment to your sex life, you might try scheduling 'sex dates' outside these times. If you and your partner both work close to home, consider meeting for a lunchtime rendezvous.

EAT YOGHURT, STARVE YEAST

After menopause, your vagina loses some of its protective lining. That means it becomes more easily abraded and more prone to bacterial and yeast infections, which cause itching, irritation and, often, pain during intercourse.

The problem is that the oral antibiotics designed to take care of the bacterial infections can also lead to more vaginal yeast infections – at a time when you're already more vulnerable. Why the complications? Oral antibiotics are formulated to fight bacteria throughout the body and, unfortunately, in the process they also annihilate the beneficial ones in the reproductive tract. As a result, the normally small, harmless population of yeast that reside in the reproductive canals can increase wildly.

To fight off yeast naturally, treat yourself to at least one large serving (about two individual pots) of yoghurt a day. Most yoghurt contains beneficial bacteria in the form of acidophilus and bifidus (often labelled as 'active cultures') that help suppress yeast. (Check the pot to make sure it lists active or live cultures.) Yoghurt with the least sugar is best since sugar seems to encourage yeast.

If yoghurt doesn't agree with you, try taking acidophilus and bifidus supplements, available as drops, powders or tablets from healthfood shops. Follow package directions for dosage. Take supplements at least two hours after the antibiotic. Otherwise, you'll risk killing off the bacteria in the supplement. If you have any serious gastrointestinal problems that require medical attention, check with your doctor before taking the supplement.

Banish Vaginal Dryness

When a woman reaches menopause and oestrogen levels are at an all-time low, the walls of her vagina may become weak, thin and dry enough to cause discomfort, especially during sex. For some, intercourse may hurt even with ample foreplay. To remedy vaginal dryness, experts offer the following advice.

Use the right lubricant. You might be tempted to reach for the petroleum jelly. Not a good idea! Petroleum jelly can break down condoms. Plus, it isn't water-soluble, so it remains in the vagina, where it can harbour yeast and other infection-producing microbes.

Instead, try a vaginal lubricant, such as Astroglide or KY Jelly, designed to relieve friction during sex by coating your vaginal walls. Unlike a moisturizer, lubricants tend to evaporate, and often need to be reapplied during intercourse.

Try an oestrogen cream. These prescription creams are applied directly into the vagina. They relieve dryness by keeping vaginal tissue moist, healthy and strong, explains Dr Brian Walsh, assistant professor of obstetrics and gynaecology and reproductive biology at Harvard Medical School. Because the hormone stays mostly in the vagina, oestrogen creams don't raise blood levels of oestrogen, making this an attractive option if you experience breakthrough bleeding or other undesirable side effects from oestrogen in tablet form.

Use a vaginal ring. The ring – about the size of a diaphragm and inserted by either you or your doctor – is kept in the vagina for up to three months, where it releases a steady, low dose of oestrogen, says Dr Walsh. Studies show that it works well to relieve both vaginal dryness and

RECLAIMING YOUR SEXUALITY

It's not unusual for a postmenopausal woman to experience a narrowing of the vagina that prevents penetration, particularly if she has spent years without a partner. Fortunately, a vaginal dilator can retrain her anatomy for a sexual relationship.

A dilator is a smooth glass wand that is inserted manually into the vagina on a daily basis for anywhere from one to six months, explains Dr Brian Walsh. In cases of severe narrowing, a patient may need to gradually increase the size of the dilator over a period of months. Once the muscles are widened, the condition will not return as long as regular intercourse is resumed.

A long hiatus from sex can also heighten the effects of the vaginal atrophy common among menopausal women. Atrophy is characterized by drying and thinning of tissues in and around the vagina, a situation that makes it prone to infection and easily irritated. To offset those symptoms, dilators are normally used in conjunction with topical oestrogen creams, which enable the vagina to produce natural secretions and improve suppleness. Both dilators and oestrogen creams are available by prescription only.

urinary tract complaints. Some women prefer the ring over creams because it's less messy.

Lubricate with liquorice. Although liquorice is better known for treating coughs and ulcers, natural healthcare professionals have found that it does wonders for toning the mucous membranes of the reproductive system as well. 'When tender vaginal tissue needs to be moistened, liquorice is a choice remedy,' according to Dr Helen Healy, a naturopathic doctor.

Unlike topically applied lubricants, which are quickly absorbed into the vaginal tissue, liquorice is believed to imitate the role of oestrogen in the body, activating the production of mucus and helping to 'plump up' the thinning vaginal wall, says Dr Healy. For that reason, it's a good remedy for women who forgo hormone replacement therapy (HRT). She suggests using only deglycyrrhizinated liquorice, labelled DGL. Whole liquorice can stimulate the adrenal glands, which aggravates hypertension and could create serious risks, especially in ageing women. Tablets marked DGL provide the benefits without those risks.

Begin by taking two 380-milligram tablets of the dried herb three times daily to keep the vaginal area moist throughout the day, she says. Once the vaginal tissue is fortified, you might find that fewer tablets are necessary. Use it as long as needed. Incidentally, if you're a fan of liquorice

CHANGE YOUR VIDEO FARE

If you're spending too many nights renting *Star Trek* videos rather than shooting off your own rockets, you and your lover might consider a more arousing form of entertainment. Films with steamy love scenes, particularly those depicting the kind of characters you can relate to, can turn up the heat for menopausal women who experience low libidos, according to Dr Barbara D. Bartlik, a psychiatrist.

Since your oestrogen and testosterone levels wane as you age, you may encounter diminished sensitivity in your breasts and genital area, often increasing the time it takes to feel sexually aroused. The bottom line is that many women require more intense forms of stimulation, and that's where erotic

sticks, don't try them – or any other liquorice sweet – instead of the liquorice tablets. Liquorice sweets contains no herbal liquorice at all.

Avoid antihistamines. The antihistamines you take to relieve your nose and eyes during the allergy season may stifle sexual comfort. That's because in addition to drying out the mucous membranes in your sinuses, these drugs also rob moisture from the lining of your vagina.

As an alternative to antihistamine drugs, consider using the nutritional supplement quercetin, a bioflavonoid derived from citrus fruit and buckwheat, suggests naturopath Dr Tori Hudson. Rather than drying out your body, quercetin goes to work on the cells that release histamines, stabilizing them and preventing such reactions as watery eyes and runny noses. Dr Hudson recommends taking 200 to 400 milligrams of quercetin three times per day, between meals, through the allergy season. Quercetin is available in tablet form from healthfood shops.

Discover Your Alluring Self

If you've been with the same man for years, you might think it's impossible to get that magic back. The thought might even make you smile. Me? Alluring to the man I've shared a bathroom with for years? Yes and yes. That's because allure isn't just a way to get a partner. It's a way to keep one.

films can help. Erotic images actually flood the body with some of the same hormones that sex does. Not only can torrid love scenes excite sexual feelings, but they can also introduce you to new, possibly more enjoyable methods for achieving fulfillment, says Dr Bartlik.

Unlike pornography, the type of film you might want to seek out, as a mature woman, is from the 'erotica' category of adult entertainment. Good erotica films feature respectable characters in sensitive, sexually charged relationships. If you're scanning the video shelves looking for a little sophistication, select films produced by women and those depicting more mature couples on the cover, says Dr Bartlik. Keep in mind also that films featuring characters with less 'model-like' bodies will help you connect to the action better than those targeted to a younger audience.

PAMPER YOURSELF CAREFULLY

Bath oils, bubbles, deodorant soaps, douches, decorative toilet tissue and even some laundry detergents can trigger discomfort in your delicate vaginal tissues – a particular concern for menopausal women, according to Dr Mary Jane Minkin, clinical professor of obstetrics and gynaecology at Yale University School of Medicine and co-author of *What Every Woman Needs to Know About Menopause.*

Before the onset of menopause, the hormone oestrogen keeps your vagina lubricated, which protects it from potentially irritating substances. But as oestrogen levels start to drop, the mucous membranes of your vagina become thinner and less moist. Soaps, which wash away your body's protective oils, only enhance that drying effect, increasing the likelihood of painful intercourse. What's more, once damaged by irritants, thin vaginal tissues are more prone to yeast and bacterial infections, another source of sexual discomfort.

Deodorant soaps, which usually contain perfumes and dyes, can be especially hard on sensitive tissue. Two milder brands that Dr Minkin recommends are Dove (white only) and Neutrogena. When it comes to baths, soaking in a tub of soapy bubbles or scented oils is an invitation for irritation. Showers are best, but oatmeal baths, or even daily baths without added soaps, are also OK.

As for laundry detergents, it's best to stick to the brand your body's used to. But if you notice irritation, switch to something non-biological, or designed for sensitive skin. Flush your affection for decorative or coloured toilet tissue as well, she says. Always use an undyed or white variety since dyes are potential irritants. And definitely don't douche, Dr Minkin says. Douching further strips your vagina of natural lubricants.

'Making an effort to look attractive to your partner is a sign of respect,' says Dr Carol Rinkleib Ellison, a clinical psychologist and sex researcher. 'It says, "You're important to me".' That said, the simplest changes are often the most dramatic. Here are some experts' favourite suggestions for enhancing your looks.

Apply some lipstick. Lipstick lights up your face. You don't have to go for vixen-red lips. Cool colours, such as cranberry and raspberry, look best on fair or ruddy skin; warm colours, such as brick and coral, on darker skin. Add lip gloss over the lipstick for moist, larger-looking lips.

Update your hairstyle. Many women wear the same hairstyle for decades, which is a big mistake. But you don't want to entrust just any stylist with your new look. Look for a salon with a well-established clientèle and a reputation for being trendy but not bizarre. To find the right stylist, look for someone who's around your age and has an attractive, updated look.

Sexier hairstyles are tousled with lots of volume. But ideally your style should also be low-maintenance and loose enough so that you (or your partner!) can run your fingers through it.

Ignore the scales. Just because you might be carrying a bit more weight than you'd like doesn't necessarily mean you're less alluring. (In fact, your partner might appreciate your curvy, womanly figure a *lot* more than you do. Ask him!) You just have to flatter your proportions. If you have larger hips, for example, balance your silhouette with shoulder pads. Avoid skirts and trousers with pleats, and dress in one colour.

Flaunt your assets. The greatest beauty secret of all is to work with what you have – and then work it. If you've always been told that you have beautiful hands, treat yourself to a weekly manicure and call attention to your hands with beautiful rings. If he has always loved your breasts, accentuate them with exquisite bras and scoop-neck tops and jumpers.

(Un)Dress for Success

Sexy lingerie really can add spice to your sex life – and we guarantee that it will get his interest. So . . . are you ready to graduate from plain white briefs and a bra? As with tops or shoes, you may not know what you want until you try it on. But it always helps to have some idea of what you're looking for. Is it elegant or racy, or somewhere in between? Which features do you want to accentuate? What's your psychological comfort level? Here are some ideas to help you choose your new undercover look.

Go on a lingerie safari. Wander through department and lingerie stores and see what catches your eye. Bright colours or dark jewel tones? Silk and satin, or lace and feathers? Styles that cover, or that reveal? Whatever you choose, you should feel emotionally comfortable in it, but it should also give you a feeling of excitement and anticipation.

Accentuate the positives. Lingerie should always accentuate the body part you're most proud of while it downplays flaws. If you're big all over, try a full-length silk or satin gown (perhaps with strategically placed lace, ties or cutaways). If you have heavy hips and thighs, avoid thongs, and choose a knee-length gown or a short style that comes to just above the knees. And if you're small-chested, don't think that bustiers are only for the well-endowed – many women with a small bust can look great in a bustier (or one of the many new water- and air-filled push-up bras designed to amplify your curves).

Pick the right colour. Colour sends a message. If you want to play innocent, wear white or soft pink. If you want to be the harlot, wear red or leopard-patterned. If you're not sure, go with classic black or a jewel tone.

Add sexy heels. High-heeled shoes make any woman's legs look longer and thinner.

Indulge in Herbal Aphrodisiacs

Herbalists say that you can recapture that 'swept away' feeling with the help of herbal potions, oils and teas. Here are the details on the passion-producing botanicals that can help the most.

Breathe in a sensual aroma. If you want to subtly perfume the air with sensuality and create a passionate atmosphere, there are several essential oils to consider.

Rose and amber have long associations with love and sensuality, and some say the scent of sandalwood can make you feel very centred in your body, very aware of physical sensation. Just add a few droplets of your chosen essential oil to a cup of warm water (the heat will release the aroma). But don't drink it by mistake!

Take massage to new heights. Just a few drops of the same essential oils, when added to an ounce of jojoba oil, can bring new sensual dimensions to a full-body massage before lovemaking. Massage each other from head to toe. Concentrate first on relaxation by working on tense spots such as the upper back, then let your touch become slower, more caressing, even arousing. Include erogenous zones like the backs of the knees and the inner thighs.

Drink some damiana. The Mexican herb damiana has a widely established folk reputation for enlivening the feminine libido, explains David Winston, a herbalist. Experts don't agree on whether or not it's consistently an aphrodisiac, but the herb is generally accepted for its ability to stabilize your emotions. Because of the herb's mild mood-enhancement abilities, Winston recommends damiana when he hears women complain of low libido. The theory is that since the herb can curb your anxiety levels and lift you out of the doldrums, your lovin' feelings have more chance to flourish. To make a quick damiana tea, pour boiling water over dried damiana leaves in a cup and let them steep for ten minutes.

For more hints on lifting your libido, see page 201.

Sex and Chronic Disease

Couples living with a major illness, such as heart disease or cancer, often struggle with sexual problems. Sometimes they give up on sex entirely. And that's too bad because our sexual feelings and our need for physical closeness don't end when we get ill. If anything, they become more important.

At the same time, it's not fair to expect that a major health problem will have no effect on a couple's sexuality or level of intimacy. So what follows is a condition-by-condition guide to four major health problems, all of which can be experienced by menopausal and postmenopausal women. It explains how each can affect sexuality and offers practical ways to express sexual feelings that don't necessarily involve intercourse.

Arthritis: Go for a Good Soak

In the most common form of arthritis, known as osteoarthritis, the cartilage that covers the ends of bones degenerates, causing bone to rub against bone. This friction causes pain and swelling of the joints, most commonly in the hips, knees and back. This pain and swelling also limit flexibility, which can make sex difficult.

Not surprisingly, many women with arthritis lose interest in sex, and it's not hard to see why. Being in physical pain doesn't naturally lead most of us to erotic thoughts.

If possible, treat yourself (and your mate) to a hot tub. Water's soothing warmth and buoyancy can relieve joint pain and stiffness. (It's also an ideal place to cuddle, talk or mess around.) If you have lung or heart disease, diabetes or high or low blood pressure, or have undergone joint replacement, don't use a hot tub without asking your doctor first.

If you never seem to feel in the mood, talk to your doctor. Common arthritis medications, such as prednisone and muscle relaxants, can affect sex drive and the ability to climax. You may be able to take another medication that works just as well but doesn't dampen your libido.

And finally, don't let a negative body image cheat you out of sex. To feel better about your body, pamper it. Take scented bubble baths. Sleep on satin sheets. Treat yourself to a massage. (Ask your partner if he might serve as your masseur.) And if your doctor says it's OK, get regular exercise. Working out often makes people feel stronger, both physically and mentally.

Cancer: Try a Little Kama Sutra

Being diagnosed with cancer – and living with it – can be emotionally devastating. Understandably, both men and women can experience an emotional shutdown that kills sexual desire. To complicate matters, cancer treatments can affect desire and performance. If a woman's ovaries are surgically removed or are damaged by chemotherapy, for example, the resulting sudden loss of oestrogen can cause her vagina to become dry and tight, one symptom of sudden menopause.

If lovemaking in the missionary position hurts, experiment with other positions that let you control the movement. The woman-on-top position, for example, often works well. Or you and your partner can try lying on your sides, either face-to-face or in a 'spooning' position. If you have had a mastectomy and aren't ready to expose the scar during intercourse, consider wearing a brief nightgown or a camisole, or a bra with a prosthesis inside.

Above all, it's especially important to be patient and flexible with each other. It seems obvious, but when you feel angry, sad or vulnerable, share those feelings with your partner. While the things you used to do in bed may no longer be possible or practical, learning to express and respond to negative feelings can strengthen your trust in each other, which can increase intimacy and make it easier to be sexually playful.

Heart Disease: Start Small

When we're aroused, our hearts beat faster and we breathe more rapidly. That's why many people still mistakenly believe that sex is a no-no for anyone with a heart problem. And while studies do suggest that women with heart disease may be more depressed and take longer to resume sexual activity than men, it's really common only in films for people to have heart attacks during sex. In fact, if either of you is depressed, tender touching may actually make you feel better.

Nonetheless, according to one estimate, between 50 and 75 per cent of men and women who have had heart attacks drastically cut down on sex or avoid it completely. In order to reclaim your sex life, start with the small gestures. Take the pressure off intercourse and instead focus on holding, kissing or caressing each other. Discover other ways to give and receive pleasure, such as mutual massage or oral sex.

If you take the prescription heart drug glyceryl trinitrate for chest pain associated with exertion, your doctor will probably suggest that you take it shortly before sex to stave off the pain of an angina attack. If you take other drugs, pay attention to how they may affect your sex drive or performance. If either of you seems impaired by prescriptions, your doctor may be able to switch you to a different, yet still effective, drug.

Osteoporosis: Take It from the Top

Sex can't be gratifying if it means putting painful pressure on frail bones threatened or damaged by osteoporosis. In the advanced stages of the disease, the bones in your spine can become so weak that they break, literally, with a sneeze. These fractures are painful and take a long time to heal. What's more, bones elsewhere in your body are also more fragile and susceptible to breaks, especially the hips and wrists.

Therefore, having sex while lying on your back with the full weight of your partner on top can be both dangerous and painful if you have brittle bones. But just because the missionary position is uncomfortable does not mean that you have to take a vow of celibacy. Rather, taking the lead in sex will ensure your safety and comfort.

Climbing on top could take you back into the pleasure zone. 'If you

want to avoid pain, the woman-on-top position may help because you have more control,' explains Dr Domeena C. Renshaw, a psychologist and expert in sexual dysfunction.

The most basic method is to lie over your partner; this is called a reverse missionary position when the woman is on top. Or you can sit up and straddle his pelvis (unless, of course, you have knee pain). In that case, continue to experiment with positions where you are on top. Dr Renshaw reminds couples to maintain a sense of humour and adventure about testing new positions, and to communicate about what feels pleasurable for both.

The most important thing to remember about sex and menopause is this: it ain't over yet. If you keep an open mind and make the effort to engage your partner, you may find postmenopausal sex to be the best sex of your life. (After all, there are no periods, no birth control and no kids in the house!) Enjoy yourself. You deserve it.

PART
3

Menopause Symptoms and Solutions

The best way to get through the menopause is to find out everything you can about it – symptoms, treatments, options. In this section, we'll give you an overview of the symptoms you may experience and the ways to handle them, as well as the benefits and drawbacks of your treatment options. Armed with the latest information, you can make the right choices for who you are, your unique lifestyle and your menopause experience.

Chapter

7

THE MENOPAUSE SYMPTOM SOLVER

Tʜᴇ ᴍᴇɴᴏᴘᴀᴜsᴇ ᴜsʜᴇʀs ɪɴ ᴀ ʜᴏsᴛ ᴏꜰ ᴄʜᴀɴɢᴇs ᴛᴏ ʙᴏᴅʏ ᴀɴᴅ mind, some of which are admittedly difficult to ignore, such as hot flushes and weight gain. At the opposite end of the spectrum are the silent changes – such as rising blood pressure – which are frequently undetected despite their serious consequences. Somewhere in the middle lurk the easily over-looked changes that are often chalked up to everyday stress, like insomnia or anxiety.

And while the changes that menopause brings can affect the quality of your life, the extent to which they do is largely up to you – that is, if you're prepared to handle them head-on. To help you do just that, this chapter covers the most common symptoms associated with menopause in an easy-to-use A-to-Z format, beginning with Anxiety and going all the way through to Weight Gain. Just look up the symptom or symptoms that are bothering you, and we'll show you exactly what you can do to keep them from undermining your health and happiness. We've also included 'Medical Alert' boxes that warn you about problems that might require attention from your doctor.

Ready to find some answers to keep you from muddling through meno-pause? Read on, and take charge of what can be the time of your life.

ANXIETY

Rare is the woman who reaches the menopause without having lain awake her fair share of nights worrying over *something*, be it her job, a child's exams, or the grey hairs that collect in her hairbrush. But don't worry. That's normal.

'When we're confronted with problems and don't have solutions, the emotional response is anxiety,' says Dr Susan Heitler, a clinical psychologist. 'Women are especially likely to experience anxiety when they're vaguely disturbed about a problem, like having too much to do and too little time in which to do it.'

In women, hormonal fluctuations may also play a role in aggravating the anxiety response, though scientists have yet to work out how or why. They do know that women seem more prone to anxious feelings just prior to their periods as well during puberty and around menopause – times of life when hormone levels change dramatically.

The fact is that millions of us worry too much. We virtually train ourselves to worry, sometimes to the point where it brings on feelings of vulnerability, which of course only reinforces the habit. So how do you reverse the process if you've crossed the worry line?

Give yourself permission to feel anxious. Try to perceive your anxiety as an amber light, not a red one, advises Dr Heitler. 'Anxiety tells you to look at how you can deal more effectively with a potential problem. It doesn't tell you to give up on doing what you want to do.'

SIGNS AND SYMPTOMS

ANXIETY

Anxiety is often confused with fear. The difference is that with fear, you know what's frightening you and can take action. Because anxiety is dread of the not yet known, tracing your feelings to a particular problem can be difficult. Left unchecked, anxiety can lead to sleeplessness, irritability, overeating or loss of appetite and difficulty concentrating. It may also contribute to high blood pressure and heart disease.

What Can You Do?

If you are living with anxiety that amounts to more than everyday worry, prescription medication and therapy with a trained counsellor are probably in order. You can take some natural steps, however, to reduce and eliminate worry and negative stress and to minimize anxiety-related episodes.

Never worry alone. When you talk about your worries with a trusted friend, colleague or relative, the toxicity dissipates. You find solutions; your concerns aren't so overwhelming. Research shows that the more isolated we feel, the more we tend to worry.

Let the worry go. Chronic worriers have a difficult time doing this because they usually do just the opposite. They hold on as though worrying will fix the problem. It won't.

Devise an action plan. 'The very best antidote to anxiety is to gather information,' says Dr Heitler. Pull out a sheet of paper and write down exactly what is bothering you. Then review your list and note what you need to do to handle the problems. 'For example, if you're losing your job, write down your fears of not having enough money to pay bills or whether you'll find another job quickly. Perhaps you can get information from your family about loan possibilities or talk to human resources about other positions within your company,' she suggests.

Take a breather. When you feel that you are in the grip of anxious feelings, take a relaxing, cleansing breath. Close your eyes and inhale deeply from your belly. Silently repeat the word 'calm', drawing out the *m* and exhaling to a count of ten. Repeat three or four times.

Take the fantasy route. Sit down in a comfortable chair, close your eyes and picture yourself lying on a beautiful beach. Inhale and exhale deeply as you visualize yourself basking in the sunshine, listening to the ocean waves and seeing the palm trees rustling in the wind. 'Soon enough, your breathing and heart rate will slow down, your stress level will drop, your anxiety will disappear, and your thoughts will clear,' says Dr Heitler.

Avoid the superwoman trap. If you usually have 20 errands to run and household chores to do, decide which are the most important and postpone the rest. 'You may have to cut back the number of hours you spend on work, split the chores and errands with your husband, or hire some help,' says Dr Heitler.

Medical Alert

ANXIETY

If your symptoms disrupt your life, making it impossible to work, drive or simply enjoy the day without a torrent of fears and worries, see your doctor. And if feelings of anxiety are accompanied by physical symptoms, such as heart palpitations, trembling, sweating, headaches, nausea, faintness or shortness of breath, an underlying anxiety disorder may be at play. But you're not alone – more than nine million people in the UK live with an anxiety disorder, a type of medical illness that includes panic attacks, phobias, post-traumatic stress disorder, obsessive-compulsive disorder and generalized anxiety disorder. In Australia, some 15 per cent of the population suffers from an anxiety disorder, a figure that is much the same in New Zealand, South Africa, Europe and the US. Many different options for medication and forms of talk therapy exist that may help you regain a sense of normality in your day-to-day life.

Find time to have fun. Make personal time a priority. Schedule fun things on your calendar, and don't let other matters interfere – even if it means leaving your job on time or saying no to another obligation.

'At the end of the workday, make it a point to leave your job emotionally as well as physically. When you get home, order a takeaway and relax by lying down and listening to music, reading or playing with the dog or cat,' says Dr Heitler. It's essential to good health that we make time to relax and unwind.

The good thing about feeling anxious is that it's a barometer, giving you feedback on what's going on in your life. 'So listen to your anxious feelings and begin shortening your to-do list to a manageable size,' she says. (Find more on moods on page 243.)

BREAST PAIN AND LUMPS

Breast pain is so common that just about every woman will experience it at some point in her life. And because women tend to fear breast cancer more than any other disease, it's understandable that 'Is it cancer?' is the first question we typically ask. Fortunately, breast pain is rarely a symptom of breast cancer and often resolves on its own.

Hormonal changes or premenstrual water retention, which tend to occur in both breasts, may be to blame since pain and swelling usually correspond to the menstrual cycle. Sometimes, tender fluid-filled cysts or benign lumps develop in the milk glands, leading to fibrocystic breast disease. This common cyclical condition, which is not really a disease, is caused by accumulated fluid and strands of fibrous tissue. Other, non-cyclical causes of breast pain include trauma, infection and injury.

If you're not sure why you have breast pain, try keeping a daily diary for a month or two and see if the pain comes and goes with your menstrual cycle. Note also the degree to which it interferes with your daily life.

Then see your doctor to request a clinical breast exam. Ask to have a mammogram, if needed, to rule out a more serious cause for your pain and inflammation – not to mention for your own peace of mind. Not all doctors will oblige, but if you are concerned, it's worth finding a sympathetic doctor who can arrange an examination. For persistent breast pain, ask your doctor about taking the prescription medication danazol (Danol).

For more on reducing breast cancer risk, see page 233.

What Can You Do?

Assuming that your doctor has assured you that you have nothing serious to worry about, here is what experts suggest to relieve breast pain and perhaps even reduce the lumpiness on your own.

Strike oil. Evening primrose oil is an anti-inflammatory that can relieve tenderness and help shrink breast cysts. It is rich in gamma-

---

SIGNS AND SYMPTOMS

BREAST PAIN AND LUMPS

Breast pain and inflammation are more common in younger women who are still menstruating than in postmenopausal women. Discomfort ranges from mild tenderness in some women to excruciating pain in others.

linolenic acid, an essential fatty acid, and is available over-the-counter. Try taking two 500-milligram capsules a day to start – but no more than six a day. For some women, it can take several months to experience relief.

Cut the caffeine. Coffee, tea, cola and chocolate contain methylxanthines, naturally occurring substances that may contribute to a fibrocystic breast problem.

Pop extra E. Some studies have shown that taken in significant doses, vitamin E can prevent breast lumps from returning, though the results are mixed. Nonetheless, many people swear by this remedy, and some experts think it may be because vitamin E encourages your body to get rid of the excess oestrogen that seems to aggravate sensitive breast tissue. Take 400 to 600 IU a day. (Get your doctor's go-ahead first.)

Feast on fibre. Build your diet around plant foods such as fruit, vegetables, pulses and wholegrain bread, pasta and cereals. A low-fat, high-fibre diet lowers oestrogen levels, which means less lumpiness and discomfort.

Wrap them in ginger. This pungent herb is a powerful anti-inflammatory that will relieve the soreness and reduce swelling, says Mindy Green, founder of the American Herbalists Guild and director of education services for the Herb Research Foundation. Grate four tablespoons of the fresh herb. Sprinkle the shavings evenly on a thin cloth. Fold in half. Then wet it with hot water. Apply to each breast for 10 to 20 minutes. Repeat two or three times a day, if possible.

If using powdered ginger (the kind found in your spice rack) is more convenient, add one teaspoon of powdered ginger to 480 ml (16 fl oz) of hot water. Dip a flannel in the solution and apply it to your skin.

If you have sensitive skin, rub some vegetable oil on your breasts before applying the ginger compress. The oil may help to prevent your skin from turning red and overheating.

Soothe with castor oil. Castor oil is great for relieving tenderness and breaking up fibrous tissue, says Mindy.

Dip a dry flannel in some castor oil and apply it to your breasts. Place a hot-water bottle on top of the flannel for 20 to 30 minutes. Or rub the castor oil directly onto your breasts. Cover them with clingfilm and a thin towel. Place a hot-water bottle on top for the same amount of time.

> **Medical Alert**
> ## BREAST PAIN AND LUMPS
>
> See your doctor if your breast pain continues every month despite self-treatment. You should also see your doctor if you notice:
>
> - Breast pain that comes on suddenly, especially when you haven't been experiencing monthly pain
> - Breast pain that occurs after you start a new drug or hormone replacement therapy
> - Bloody or milky discharge from one or both nipples
> - Any breast lump or thickening, whether or not it is painful

Wear a supportive bra. The mere act of not wearing a bra can contribute to breast pain since the weight of the breasts can cause discomfort. So, for many women, wearing a supportive bra is helpful. Be sure you wear a bra that's constructed in a way that won't add to the irritation. Look inside the cups and make sure that there are no seams and that nothing is pushing up against you. If there is an underwire, make sure that it's very well-padded so that it doesn't add to the friction. Sports bras usually fit all of these criteria.

DEPRESSION

Women are three times more likely than men to develop depression. In addition, 'Women have times in their lives when they seem especially vulnerable to depression,' says Dr Laura Epstein Rosen, an expert in family therapy. Sometimes the risk is biologically driven, as when hormone levels fluctuate just after childbirth and just before menopause. Other times it is externally driven – perhaps by the death of a parent, divorce, job loss or some other major life event.

Even everyday conflict can brew into mild depression, says Dr Susan Heitler, a clinical psychologist. 'When you want x and your partner wants y, you have a problem,' she explains. If you repeatedly give up what you want

---

SIGNS AND SYMPTOMS

DEPRESSION

Mild depression often manifests itself as deeply negative feelings of sorrow, guilt, discouragement and powerlessness. More severe cases may be accompanied by symptoms such as loss of appetite, lack of sleep and difficulty concentrating. (See page 243 for more on mood disorders.)

---

so that your partner gets what he wants, without seeking a mutually satisfying compromise, you may pay an emotional price in the long run.

The good news about depression is that once you recognize that you have it, you can treat it. 'By knowing when you are vulnerable to depression and by recognizing its signs and symptoms, you can get the help you need,' says Dr Rosen.

What's more, depression may draw your attention to some aspect of your life that needs evaluation and change, says Dr Margaret Jensvold, director of the Institute for Research on Women's Health. 'If you find yourself repeatedly getting upset or sad about the same situation, you need to come to terms with that situation, one way or another,' she advises.

What Can You Do?

For severe depression, you need to see a doctor, who may recommend a combination of talk therapy and antidepressant drugs. Mild depression responds well to self-care measures like these.

Illuminate yourself. 'Before we use any herbs or supplements, we need to find out what's causing the depression,' says Dr Ellen Kamhi, author of *Cycles of Life: Herbs and Energy Techniques for Women*. Sometimes it's something relatively simple, such as lack of sunlight, which can be treated with a light box.

Light treatment should be considered even before using herbs, she says, because there are no chemicals or toxicities in light, and you can operate a light box at work or home. Use this treatment only in consultation with your doctor, who can explain proper use of the box and set up an appropriate treatment schedule.

Eat small meals every two or three hours. Sticking with a regular mini-meal schedule helps keep your blood sugar on a more even keel. 'For some people, low blood sugar can trigger depression,' says Dr Jensvold. Of course, you should make sure that each mini-meal is well-balanced. Choose healthy foods such as whole grains, fruit, vegetables and fat-free or low-fat dairy products.

Grab your partner. A study published in the *Journal of Nervous and Mental Disease* found that having a supportive spouse and other positive relationships reduced the likelihood of major depression.

Move for your mood. Physical activity is a great way to prevent and treat depression. Researchers don't know exactly why exercise helps, but they suggest it may enhance our sense of mastery so we feel more mentally and physically in control. Aerobic activity may also help vent pent-up frustration. And mood-enhancing endorphins (those brain chemicals responsible for the phenomenon known as 'runner's high') released during exercise could also be involved. Aim for at least 30 minutes of exercise most days. If you want, you can break it into three sets of ten minutes each.

Expand your exercise horizons. Yoga and t'ai chi are excellent depression remedies. For one thing, if you take a class, you'll bond with others, says Dr Kamhi. Also, some movements and breathing exercises in yoga and t'ai chi can stimulate glands to release mood-enhancing hormones.

Medical Alert

DEPRESSION

See your doctor if you have suicidal thoughts or have had a distinct period during which you felt down and unhappy or unable to enjoy life and have experienced any of the following symptoms for two weeks or longer. You may have severe depression, which requires professional care.

- Appetite or weight changes
- Sleep problems
- Excessive fatigue
- Excessive agitation or lethargy
- Guilty feelings
- Slow thinking or indecisiveness

FATIGUE

Fatigue is such a broad term that it can mean many different things to different people. To women facing menopause, being tired may mean that they can't lift a finger to wash another dish, while for others it means that they're so grumpy that they want to sit in their cars and scream. Still others define it as not being able to get out of bed in the morning.

Understandably, such variety in meaning makes it difficult to use in diagnosing an illness. One way to help measure fatigue, however, is to consider its relation to time. Once you've determined how long your fatigue has been around, start asking other specific questions, such as what activities make you feel most tired, whom are you with when you feel tired, and how does being tired feel. This information is vitally important to your doctor, who may be able to help you resolve the problem without any further treatment.

Acute fatigue – that is, lasting less than one month – is often easier to diagnose because chances are you know the cause. If you have the flu, for example, you probably wouldn't even mention a concern about fatigue to your doctor because you know why you're so tired. Prolonged fatigue typically lasts one to six months. Often, women who are depressed will have this type of fatigue – it develops not overnight but over a couple of months of worry, sadness, stress or sleepless nights. Another fatiguing condition that can come on gradually is hypothyroidism, in which the thyroid doesn't produce enough of its hormone, resulting in low energy levels. If you don't seek help for these conditions, you may stray into chronic fatigue territory, more than six months of exhaustion.

SIGNS AND SYMPTOMS

FATIGUE

Fatigue is a feeling of tiredness all too familiar to most people. The problem is so common that doctors estimate about one out of every ten people (many of them women) may be troubled by daytime fatigue. In fact, eight out of ten people who are referred to sleep specialists don't have trouble getting to sleep – they have trouble staying awake.

Chronic fatigue is definitely not something you should try to cope with on your own since it could reflect a serious health concern, cautions Dianne Delva, associate professor of family medicine at Queen's University, Ontario. For instance, chronic fatigue could be a sign of type 2 diabetes. Left untreated, it could lead to kidney or heart disease, blindness, stroke or other health problems.

What Can You Do?

Prolonged and chronic fatigue require a doctor's care. But to help reverse short bouts of fatigue, try these natural energy-boosting strategies.

Eat early. The sooner you eat, the better. But if you just can't face food first thing in the morning, make sure you sit down to a nutritious meal within three hours. Breakfast helps your body rev up after sleeping and helps prevent you from eating too much lunch, which can sap energy in the afternoon.

At mid-day, focus on protein. The amino acid tyrosine, supplied by high-protein food, synthesizes more of the brain's alertness chemicals and keeps the brain from manufacturing the neurotransmitter serotonin, which slows you down.

Cut caffeine after 4.30 pm. Since caffeine keeps you alert for up to six hours, it can prevent you from getting to sleep at a regular time if you consume it in the evening. That's *all* sources of caffeine, by the way – including chocolate, cola and tea.

Drink water. Aim for eight 240-ml (8-fl oz) glasses of water every day. Dehydration can cause your performance to flag measurably. Keeping a ready supply of water nearby throughout the day will encourage you to drink as much as you need, when you need it. Try leaving a water bottle on your desk or taking it with you in the car.

Treat yourself. Sometimes energy levels slump not because of how much you do but because of how much energy you expend on behalf of everyone but yourself. So, give yourself a prescription to do something for yourself today – take a half day off and do something just for you!

Take a walk. Just 20 minutes of walking, ideally after breakfast or lunch, will buoy your energy levels for as much as eight hours afterwards.

Medical Alert

FATIGUE

If you have experienced fatigue for longer than a month, see a doctor.

But don't exercise too close to bedtime because you may be too energized to fall asleep.

Don't spend too much time in bed. Sleeping too much can make you feel more, rather than less, fatigued, says Dr Alexander C. Chester, a clinical professor of medicine. Most people need seven to eight hours of sleep a night, no more.

Count the hours in your day. If you're like many women, you may have an unrealistic idea of how long it takes to perform your daily chores, and you might be trying to accomplish more than is humanly possible – which only leaves you exhausted.

To take stock, write down everything that you do each day. Next to each task, estimate how much time each task truly takes. Don't leave anything out, from the moment you rise until bedtime. Then add up the hours. If you're trying to do 23 hours' worth of work in 16 waking hours, give yourself a reality check, adjust your efforts and concentrate on doing just one thing at a time.

FRACTURES

Throughout our lives, our bones break down and rebuild in a carefully balanced process. Because the body needs small amounts of calcium circulating in the blood to help with muscle contraction and blood clotting, it frees up calcium by creating small holes in bones. To keep things in balance, the holes are then quickly repaired. Each year, 10 to 30 per cent of your skeleton goes through this bone breakdown and rebuilding – but the process changes as we age, and we no longer rebuild bone as quickly as it is broken down.

The result of this imbalance? On average, we lose one-third of our bone in the first five years after menopause, when our ovaries stop producing the oestrogen that keeps bone loss to a minimum. And although we still get oestrogen from body fat, skin and muscle after menopause, it's not enough to significantly protect against bone loss.

Unless we take protective measures, this bone loss can advance to osteoporosis, a disease in which the bones become fragile and fracture easily. In fact, one in two women will fracture a bone because of the disease.

What Can You Do?

Bone loss may be inevitable, but osteoporosis isn't. Too often, it is dismissed as a normal part of ageing, but it's completely preventable. 'Osteoporosis should never happen,' says Dr Nancy DiMarco, a professor of nutrition and food sciences.

Most women know that calcium and weight-bearing exercise lower their risk of osteoporosis, but there's much more you can do to protect your bones. 'I'm always surprised when women who say they exercise and take calcium think that's all they have to do,' says Dr Jane Lukacs.

Don't stop there. Find out other ways to slow bone loss.

Count your calcium. Our bodies need to maintain about 1 kg (2.2 lb) of calcium to keep bones healthy. But compared with younger women, women aged 65 and older are able to absorb less than half the calcium they consume.

SIGNS AND SYMPTOMS

FRACTURES

After age 50, half of all Western women have bones weak enough to fracture. And unfortunately for many, a fracture may be the first sign that osteoporosis has set in because there are virtually no outward symptoms before then.

Osteoporosis-related fractures commonly occur in the vertebrae, wrist, hip or forearm from surprisingly minor activities, such as bending over, lifting, jumping or tripping. Once the disease progresses, just opening a door can result in broken bones.

Between the ages of 19 and 50, you need at least 1,000 milligrams of calcium a day. That's about 3½ glasses of milk, Dr DiMarco says. After 50, aim for 1,200 milligrams, just half a glass more.

Eating dairy products, especially milk, is the best way to get calcium, Dr DiMarco says, because they provide the most concentrated and absorbable form of calcium. Women who are lactose intolerant can usually handle a small amount of milk at a time – between 125 and 250 ml (4–8 fl oz) – without feeling sick, she adds.

If you don't like milk, there are plenty of other ways to get calcium, especially with the number of calcium-fortified foods on the rise. But don't go overboard. Try not to get more than 2,400 milligrams of calcium a day. Any amount over 2,400 milligrams may not be absorbed.

Drink tea. Women, especially postmenopausal ones, who drink two or more cups of coffee a day have reduced bone density because coffee increases calcium loss in urine.

Tea, on the other hand, has isoflavonoids, plant compounds that help our bones. A study of postmenopausal women in the UK found that drinking at least one cup of tea a day increased the drinkers' bone density by about five per cent, compared with the bone density of women who didn't drink tea. Those who added milk had an even higher bone density.

Researchers think that isoflavonoids' ability to mimic oestrogen helps maintain bone density in women after menopause.

Stop smoking. Do this, and you lower your risk of osteoporosis while you get rid of your smoker's cough. Women who smoke may have lower oestrogen levels than women who don't, and they go through menopause two years earlier.

Drink moderately. Having seven or more alcoholic drinks a week increases your risk of falls and hip fractures. Alcohol also lowers your body's ability to build bone. Further, many women who drink too much alcohol have poor nutrition habits, says Dr Robert Marcus, an endocrinologist at Stanford University.

Fall-proof your house. If you've received a low score on a bone-mass screening, then a short fall for you could lead to a fracture, so take precautions around your home and in daily activities. Wear shoes that are appropriate for the surface you are walking on. Remove slippery carpets from

Medical Alert

FRACTURES

Fortunately, bone density tests can reveal signs of osteoporosis before breaks occur. Review the following list of risk factors and talk to your doctor about what type of screening is right for you.

- Thin and small-boned frame
- Irregular menstrual periods or fewer than ten cycles a year
- History of eating disorders
- Family history of osteoporosis
- Generalized bone pain and tenderness
- Smoking
- History of taking corticosteroids, anticonvulsants such as phenytoin (Epanutin), thyroid medication or blood thinners.

your home, and keep electrical cords tucked out of the way. Watch where you walk, especially if the surfaces, such as streets and pavements, are uneven.

You'll find medical options for osteoporosis on page 244.

HAIR LOSS

Men worry when they go bald. Some grow their remaining hair longer in the front or on one side and then comb it to cover their bare domes. Some even get toupées. But no matter how they cope, they have millions of other men with whom to share their pain.

Baldness is a different story for women. We're not *supposed* to go bald. 'And with all the research that's gone into male-pattern baldness, the issue in women has been relatively ignored,' says Dr Ellen W. Seely, an endocrinologist.

Most balding in women is caused by a condition known as androgenic alopecia (AGA) – the same condition that causes the majority of male baldness. Those of us with thinning hair can blame our genes, for one. 'Many women with this problem had grandmothers who had it, and

---

SIGNS AND SYMPTOMS

HAIR LOSS

It's normal to lose 100 scalp hairs a day, but you have to lose much more, over 50 per cent of your scalp hair, before the loss is noticeable. And that's just what happens to about 40 per cent of women – they notice that their hair has thinned by the time they reach menopause.

---

great-grandmothers who had it,' says Dr Seely. But we can also blame our hormones. Testosterone, for one. Too much (in men or women) means that we're more likely to lose the hair on our heads yet *grow* hair on other parts of our bodies.

A woman with this problem will go bald in the same places as her husband, such as on her temples and the top of her head, but grow hair on her chin, under her belly button, and on her inner thighs and lower back. This unusual kind of hair growth or loss could also indicate a medical problem other than AGA, so it should be checked out by an endocrinologist, says Dr Seely.

Oestrogen, on the other hand, *prolongs* the hair follicle's growth period. 'So with more oestrogen, the hair can grow longer, and there's more hair on the scalp,' says Dr Seely. This explains why women experience some hair loss after childbirth and menopause, when oestrogen levels are falling. It also explains why we can grow our hair longer than most men.

If you're concerned about baldness, first make sure that there isn't a medical issue. 'Tumours can make male hormone, which can cause baldness,' Dr Seely says. Apart from that, hair is dependent on your stress levels and diet. 'So avoiding major stresses and getting enough vitamins can help,' she says.

What Can You Do?

Given the number of factors that can cause temporary and long-term hair loss, it's difficult to know what to do. Treatments that have been reported to work in some studies include exotic herbs, amino acids and a soft laser scalp massage. Before looking into these more involved therapies, read on. You might find number of solutions that will work for you.

Relax. If you've just gone through a divorce, a move or some other major stress, your hair loss might be stress-related. Major stress can cause your roots to close down and rest for three months.

Think about other changes. If your hair is coming out in patches but you haven't experienced any major life stresses, think about the other changes in your life.

Have you started taking a new medication or changed your eating habits? Anti-thyroid drugs, anti-convulsants, diuretics and even ibuprofen can trigger hair loss in some people.

Ease up on hair treatments. Don't perm, straighten or colour your hair until it's back to normal. Chemical treatments can inflame and irritate your scalp.

Adopt an easygoing style. Give your hair a break from tight plaits and rollers, which can break hair and exaggerate thinning.

Use what men use. Apply minoxidil, a hair-restoring treatment (marketed as Regaine), to your scalp twice a day. It has been proved effective, especially for the 25 to 30 per cent of women who lose their hair because of heredity factors.

Have patience. Nothing restores hair loss in six weeks. Experts say it usually takes six months for the process to turn around.

Medical Alert
HAIR LOSS

If you have no idea why you're losing your hair, consult your doctor, who can refer you to a dermatologist who deals with hair problems. It's better to stop the process as soon as possible instead of waiting for years because it usually becomes more difficult to treat hair loss over time.

HIGH BLOOD PRESSURE

Thanks to oestrogen, high blood pressure (or hypertension) hits women later in life than it does men. Not that this female hormone's protection is iron-clad. Women can – and do – develop high blood pressure before oestrogen production wanes at menopause.

Doctors take two measurements when they check your blood pressure. The first is called the systolic reading. It indicates how hard your heart pumps to push blood through your arteries. The second, called the diastolic reading, shows how much your arteries put up resistance to the blood flow. Blood pressure is measured in millimetres of mercury, or mm Hg, and a reading of about 120 mm Hg systolic and 80 mm Hg diastolic is considered healthy. We read that simply as 120/80.

Everyone's blood pressure varies widely throughout the day. Generally, it will rise when you're exercising and drop when you're asleep. But when your baseline, or resting, reading creeps up to 140/90, you have borderline high blood pressure. That means your heart is working too hard to pump blood, either because your arteries have narrowed or stiffened with plaque or because you have too much blood in your system on account of water retention or other problems.

'If you're borderline hypertensive, there's a lot you can do to either prevent the need for drugs or reduce the amount of drugs you have to take,' says Dr Thomas Pickering, a cardiologist and professor of medicine, and author of *Good News about High Blood Pressure*.

SIGNS AND SYMPTOMS
HIGH BLOOD PRESSURE

Blood pressure normally fluctuates from day to day and even from minute to minute, depending upon activity, posture, temperature, diet, drugs and a person's emotional and physical states. But odds are that you'd never know it unless you took your blood pressure throughout the day. That's one reason high blood pressure is so dangerous – it's a symptomless disease.

What Can You Do?

Uncontrolled high blood pressure increases your risk of heart disease, kidney failure and stroke. But for most women, elevated blood pressure can be controlled before it has a chance to do any permanent harm. Here's how to get a handle on hypertension.

Have it tested. There's only one way to know for sure if you have high blood pressure – ask your doctor to check it. Once a year should be sufficient, unless your doctor orders more tests. It's a quick, painless procedure. The doctor puts an inflatable cuff around your arm and checks your pulse with a stethoscope. If you show a borderline-high reading, the doctor may order several retests over a couple of weeks or months.

Stop smoking. Smoking markedly increases your risk of developing a stroke or blood vessel damage from high blood pressure. It also encourages your body to deposit cholesterol within your coronary arteries. This decreases the size of your vessels and forces your heart to work harder. Anyone with high blood pressure should stop smoking immediately.

Eat more fish and less fat. In a study conducted in Australia, overweight men and women who ate 100 g (4 oz) of fish a day dropped six blood pressure points in four months. But those who ate fish *and* cut back on dietary fat got extra blood pressure-lowering benefits. For women who have elevated blood pressure, Dr Pickering recommends three to seven fish meals a week – more than the usual, twice-a-week directive.

Cook with garlic and basil. A cornerstone of Mediterranean cuisine, garlic has a documented blood pressure–lowering effect. Try to eat a clove or two each day. Fresh basil leaves also help keep blood pressure in check. Think pesto.

Fill up on fibre and shun processed wheat. Dietary fibre has clear cardiovascular benefits. Processed wheat, on the other hand, creates an insulin surge, which triggers a rise in blood pressure for several hours. One study, at Tulane University in New Orleans, found that subjects with the highest blood insulin levels were three times more likely to have high blood pressure. So substitute fibre-rich unprocessed wholegrain bread for that white bread to reap the benefits of the former while avoiding the harm of the latter.

Medical Alert

HIGH BLOOD PRESSURE

Your blood pressure readings ideally should be below 120/80 millimetres of mercury (mm Hg), although readings as high as 130/85 are considered normal. If your blood pressure consistently creeps above that mark, you need to start watching it carefully. A reading of 140/90 or higher means that medical treatment is appropriate.

Consume potassium, magnesium and calcium. All three minerals help keep your blood pressure down. Even better, choose food sources over supplements. 'Getting these minerals in combination naturally from food has more of an effect than taking them individually as supplements,' says Dr Pickering. This could mean a difference of 3 to 4 mm Hg.

For potassium, eat four or five daily servings of fruit and vegetables, especially cantaloupe, baked potatoes, bananas, citrus fruit and tomatoes. You'll find the highest amounts of magnesium in almonds and pumpkin seeds. Low-fat or fat-free dairy products like milk and yoghurt provide ample calcium, but so do calcium-fortified orange juice and soya milk.

Move it and lose it. Thirty minutes of daily aerobic exercise in the morning will help lower your blood pressure for most of the day. Do it regularly, and the benefits will be permanent. Carrying a bit of extra weight? Just losing weight will lower your blood pressure. Better yet, the *combination* of losing weight and getting regular exercise can pare your pressure by 20 points.

Reduce stress and add quiet activity. Stress raises blood pressure, so eliminate what you can. For example, ask for more authority in your job; the resulting sense of control reduces stress. Insist on clarity about whom you report to; trying to please too many bosses is stressful.

Then manage the stress that's left by using relaxation techniques. In one three-month study, 20 minutes a day of meditation lowered study participants' blood pressure by 11 points. Others find success with breathing exercises, nature walks or even watching tropical fish.

HOT FLUSHES

No one knows exactly what triggers hot flushes, but they seem to be linked to the hormonal changes that occur before and during menopause. 'These changes somehow stimulate the part of the brain that controls body temperature, throwing off its usually fine-tuned control,' explains Dr Robert Freedman, an expert in behavioural medicine.

As a result, the brain signals the body to dissipate heat – in other words, to flush and sweat.

If you took your temperature during a hot flush, you wouldn't have a fever. 'But hot flushes are synchronized with your core temperature (deep inside your body), which rises and falls in a predictable pattern over a 24-hour period,' notes Dr Freedman. Things start sizzling just about the time your body reaches its peak core temperature for the day – usually late afternoon or early evening. But hot flushes can occur at any time of the day or night.

Though considered physically harmless, hot flushes can make you flustered and self-conscious. The good news about hot flushes is that they actually cool down once menopause finally arrives.

For the women in one study, the number of incendiary episodes dropped to 20 per cent of their peak frequency within four years after the onset of menopause.

SIGNS AND SYMPTOMS

HOT FLUSHES

During a hot flush, blood surges to the surface of the skin on your chest, neck and head. With this increase in blood flow comes a rise in skin temperature, a slight acceleration of heart and breathing rates, and perspiration. As the hot flush dissipates heat, your body's core temperature drops (which is why you may feel cold and clammy afterwards). The entire episode usually lasts two to five minutes.

What Can You Do?

Hot flushes may take you by surprise the first couple of times they occur. But if you are like many women, you will eventually be able to tell when one is coming on. These strategies can help you weather a hot flush and prevent it from becoming too severe.

Practise deep breathing. In one study, women who had been having 20 or more hot flushes a day reduced that number by half with the help of deep breathing, says Dr Freedman. 'This technique seems to short-circuit the arousal of the central nervous system that normally occurs in the initial stages of a hot flush,' he explains.

When you feel a hot flush creeping up on you, prepare for deep breathing by sitting up straight and loosening your belt or waistband if it feels tight. Begin by exhaling through your nose longer than you normally would. Then inhale through your nose slowly and deeply, filling your lungs from the bottom up while keeping your belly relaxed. When your chest is fully expanded, exhale slowly and deeply, as if sighing. Continue this pattern of inhaling and exhaling until the hot flush subsides.

Adjust the temperature of the room. Ideally, set the thermostat at 60°F (15°C). Simplistic as it may seem, turning down the heat or using a fan or air-conditioning is solid advice, according to Dr Freedman. 'Anything that raises body temperature even a tiny bit, such as being in a room that's too hot, can aggravate a hot flush,' he says.

Monitor your reaction to spicy foods. Garlic, ginger, chilli pepper, onions and highly acidic produce such as citrus fruit and tomatoes may fuel your hot flush fire, according to Dr Judyth Reichenberg-Ullman, a naturopathic doctor. If you tend to experience hot flushes after eating one of these foods, eliminate the food from your diet for a week or so and note if your symptoms improve.

Wean yourself off the bean. Hot caffeinated drinks are a common hot flush aggravator. But you can drink soft drinks or hot herbal tea. It's not the heat or the caffeine alone that seems to cause hot flushes, but the combination of the two.

Avoid alcohol. Alcohol causes you to flush even when you aren't in a state of hormonal upheaval. It can certainly fan the flame of hot flushes.

HOT FLUSHES

See your doctor if your hot flushes become so frequent or severe that they disrupt your daily routine. Also see your doctor if hot flushes at night (called night sweats) continue for several weeks and you are having trouble sleeping as a result.

In a study at the University of North Carolina, women who had at least one alcoholic drink a week were about 13 per cent more likely to experience hot flushes than women who never drank. 'Alcohol consumption proved to be one of the strongest lifestyle risk factors for hot flushes,' according to Dr Pamela Schwingl, senior epidemiologist at Family Health International and the study's main author.

INCONTINENCE

It's only when our bodies stop making oestrogen that we realize just how much this hormone does. Take the bladder, for instance. Oestrogen keeps the linings of the bladder and urethra (the tube that carries urine from the bladder) supple and healthy. When we stop making oestrogen, our bladder control muscles weaken, often to the point where a simple sneeze or chuckle can generate an embarrassing accident.

Researchers believe that urinary incontinence affects 30 to 60 per cent of all postmenopausal women. But the good news is that it's easily controlled and, better yet, cured, says Dr Rodney Appell, Scott Professor of Female Urology at Baylor Medical College.

Among women aged 55 and younger, stress incontinence is the most common form of urinary incontinence. Women with stress incontinence may dribble urine when they cough, laugh, lift heavy objects, exert themselves suddenly, change positions quickly – any action that increases pressure on the bladder.

Stress incontinence results from stretched and weakened pelvic floor muscles, which can result from menopausal changes and abdominal

INCONTINENCE

In women, incontinence usually takes one of two forms: if you leak urine during exercise or when you cough, laugh or sneeze, it is most likely you have stress incontinence; if you have the urge to go to the loo but can't get there in time, you probably have what is called urge incontinence. The good news is that doctors say that eight out of ten women with incontinence can be helped – if they know what to do.

surgery. These muscles, which extend from the pubic bone to the tailbone, provide hammocklike support for the bladder and uterus. Both the vagina and the urethra pass through this muscular sling. When you contract the pelvic floor muscles, you squeeze your vagina and urethra shut.

While stress incontinence gives you no advance warning of a urine leak, urge incontinence sends the signal that you have to go. Unfortunately, it leaves you no time to get to a bathroom. The bladder may release just a bit of urine, or it may spill its whole load.

With urge incontinence, some factor disrupts communication between your brain and your bladder. As a result, your brain gets the message that your bladder is full, but your bladder doesn't receive its instructions to wait until you find a toilet. Weak pelvic floor muscles may contribute to urge incontinence, but other factors – such as menopausal changes, urinary tract infections and even food irritants – probably play roles as well.

What Can You Do?

To get your bladder back on track, you need to look at a variety of lifestyle factors. Be sure to include these self-care measures in your treatment routine.

Try the Kegel cure. Kegel (pelvic floor) exercises build strength and endurance in the muscles of the bladder. Most doctors recommend them as the first-line approach in treating most types of incontinence. They can be hard to learn to do correctly, however, so if you don't see any results from the following exercises after about eight weeks, talk to your doctor about referring you to a specialist, who can offer a type of 'physiotherapy' for your pelvic muscles.

To do Kegels, you quickly contract your pelvic floor muscles (the ones that you use to control your urine stream) for one to two seconds, then relax the muscles between contractions to prevent muscle fatigue. Do ten repetitions three to five times per day. As you repeat the exercise, hold the contractions for five seconds, and gradually increase to 15 seconds three to five times daily.

When done correctly, Kegels are just as effective as surgery and medication for mild to moderate stress and urge incontinence, minus the side-effects. One study found that women who practised Kegels three times a week had the most success, even after five years.

Retrain your bladder. This technique works especially well for women with urge incontinence. Begin by allowing yourself one trip to the loo every hour for a week or two. Then for another week or two, extend the time between trips by a half hour. Continue this pattern of adding half-hour increments to your routine until you are able to hold your urine for three or four hours at a time. This exercise teaches your bladder to hold more urine and become less spastic when it is full.

Stop smoking. Women who smoke cigarettes are more than twice as likely to develop stress incontinence as women who have never smoked,

---

Medical Alert

INCONTINENCE

If home remedies don't help eliminate your incontinence, see your doctor. You should also see your doctor to rule out a more serious contributing condition if you have any of the following symptoms.

- Pain or burning upon urinating
- Voiding more than 1.5 litres (2.5 pints) of urine a day
- Blood in your urine
- Change in bowel habits
- Pain during intercourse
- Numbness or weakness in your arms or legs
- Changes in vision

according to a study performed at Virginia Commonwealth University School of Medicine. Cigarettes deliver a double whammy to your bladder. Nicotine irritates it and coughing (as most smokers do) puts pressure on it.

Drink enough fluids each day. Restricting your fluid intake won't prevent leaks. In fact, it can actually aggravate incontinence by producing concentrated urine, which is highly irritating to your bladder. Drink lots of water, and choose cranberry juice, which prevents bacteria sticking to the urinary tract walls. How do you know that you are well-hydrated? Your urine should appear clear or pale yellow.

INSOMNIA

From decades of research, sleep scientists have determined that, barring unusual circumstances, women naturally sleep between 8 and 8½ hours a day. This is 1 to 1½ hours more sleep per night than the average man requires. The irony is that women very often have less time available for sleep than men, even though they need more sleep than their male counterparts.

Just how does the sleep process work? Scientists point to a biological 'clock' that each of us has within us; this internal clock operates on a 24-hour cycle and helps your body know when to do certain things, such as ready itself for sleep. For example, about an hour or two before bedtime, the pineal gland in the brain responds to signals from the biological clock and secretes a hormone called melatonin that makes you sleepy (among other things). The same clock signals your body to slow your heart rate and

SIGNS AND SYMPTOMS

INSOMNIA

One-third of all adults can't sleep at one time or another. Over time, losing even as little as an hour or so of sleep a night leads to irritability, difficulty performing tasks well and memory loss, says Dr Virgil Wooten, associate director of the Sleep Disorders Center at Eastern Virginia Medical School.

lower your body temperature and blood pressure in anticipation of sleep. It
then reactivates these vital signs a few hours before you wake up.

Your biological clock works under the assumption that you sleep at
night. Therefore, its timing is governed by the cycles of daylight and dark-
ness. This is one reason that some people who are blind experience
insomnia. It is also why some people lose sleep if they don't get enough
light during the day or wake up too early if light streams in through their
bedroom windows. Other factors – such as drinking too much coffee or
exercising late at night or simply feeling nervous – can keep you awake,
too. In addition, as women age, they're especially prone to insomnia. Once
they turn 40, women are 40 per cent more likely to experience some
degree of insomnia, thanks to the mid-life hormonal changes that precede
menopause. A few years before and after menopause, a common cause of
insomnia is night sweats. (For practical ideas on how to manage them, see
'Night Sweats' on page 206).

What Can You Do?

For most women, occasional insomnia isn't much of a problem. But a
sleepless night can leave you less than ready for the day ahead. To prevent
future episodes of sleeplessness, follow this advice.

Take a morning walk outside. 'Light exposure during the day helps
keep your body clock regulated,' says Dr Mary A. Carskadon, professor of
psychiatry and human behaviour and head of the sleep research lab at a
leading research hospital. 'An early-morning walk in the daylight upon
rising will help promote sleep at night.'

Resist the urge to nap. Napping during the day after a sleepless
night will only throw your body clock further off balance. Instead, experts
recommend consolidating your sleep to make sure you get enough of it
at night.

De-stress your bedroom. You probably don't sleep in your office.
Conversely, experts point out, you shouldn't work in your bedroom. Your
bedroom is for two things only: sleeping and sex. So remove your computer, your office reading pile, your fax machine and even your phone, if
you can. And put your TV back in the sitting room, where it belongs.

> ***Medical Alert***
>
> # INSOMNIA
>
> If you've tried the advice presented in this section and still can't easily get to sleep or stay asleep throughout the night for a month or so, see your doctor. She may refer you to a specialist or a sleep disorders clinic for further evaluation.

Set a bedtime. Adults, just like children, need a regular bedtime, says Dr Carskadon.

'We have body clocks that synchronize our systems. Establish a set sleep and wake-up time, then stick to it every day. That tells your clock to make you sleepy at night and wakeful in the morning.'

Take a hot bath. A hot bath taken early in the evening will cause your temperature to go up and then drop more quickly when you hit the sack, so you can fall asleep more easily.

Wind down before you get into bed. Giving yourself about 45 minutes of 'quiet time' before you get into bed helps signal to your body clock that the day is done and sleep time is imminent. Listen to soft music, write a letter, read something boring – but don't do anything that winds you up (and absolutely nothing work-related).

Turn the clock to the wall. Staring at the clock makes you more tense about getting back to sleep. Instead of checking the time, concentrate on restful thoughts.

Picture some numbers. If you can't sleep, try this technique. Close your eyes and relax. Count backwards slowly from 100 to zero. As you do, visualize the numbers in some beautiful way. Maybe you see them being written by a calligrapher. Or try seeing the numbers being drawn on a huge blackboard across a giant sky. Continue until sleep overtakes you.

Don't overcompensate. Don't stay in bed for 10 or 11 hours, trying to make up for lost sleep time. If you usually need eight hours, you will just have an extra two hours to toss and turn. You won't get more sleep, say the experts. And if you extend your sleep time too much, you may begin to wake up too early in the morning. It is more important to get the sleep you need on a regular basis.

IRREGULAR PERIODS AND FLOODING

Your cycles used to be regular, but now they're not. You used to know roughly how many tampons or pads you'd use during each period, but now you haven't got a clue. Nothing about your period is as it used to be.

If you're like a lot of women, you wonder whether this new irregularity is a normal part of perimenopause – or if it's a sign that something sinister is going on. More than likely, bleeding irregularities that begin in your forties or fifties – or even as early as your thirties – can be traced to the beginnings of menopause, says Susun S. Weed, a herbalist. To distinguish normal from abnormal changes, keep records. You may find that there's a certain regularity to your irregularity. If your periods are indeed erratic or profuse, consult your doctor.

What Can You Do?

Sometimes natural remedies can even out irregular menses; sometimes they can't. Our experts suggest:

Turn to agnus castus. Although it's slow to act, agnus castus tincture (also called vitex or chasteberry) is highly recommended for women who are bothered by menopausal irregularities. Susun recommends a dropperful in a small glass of water or juice two or three times a day for six to eight weeks after every irregular period.

Take a hip-swinging stroll. Walking stimulates the pelvic region and gets fluids moving through the area, so it reduces pelvic congestion, says Dr Mary Bove, a naturopathic doctor and director of the Brattleboro Naturopathic Clinic. 'I tell women to work on their pelvises, letting their hips lead their stroke as they walk, letting their hips and arms swing freely

---

SIGNS AND SYMPTOMS

IRREGULAR PERIODS AND FLOODING

As they approach menopause, many women report changes to their menstrual cycles that include either lighter or heavier bleeding, and longer, shorter or skipped periods. In most cases, there is no need for concern.

so that the whole body has a chance to stretch out.' A daily 20-minute walk will decrease the likelihood of cramps, reduce them if you have them, and brighten your mood, she says.

Savour some cinnamon. Cinnamon bark invigorates the blood, helps regulate the menstrual cycle and checks flooding, says Susun Weed. For heavy bleeding, take five to ten drops of tincture once or twice a day, or chew on a cinnamon stick. You can also simply sprinkle ground cinnamon freely on food, she advises.

Visit a lady. In a clinical study, five to ten drops of lady's mantle tincture controlled menstrual haemorrhage in virtually all of the 300 women who participated, says Susun. When taken after flooding began, lady's mantle took three to five days to become effective. When taken for one to two weeks before menstruation, it prevented flooding. She suggests using five to ten drops of the fresh plant tincture three times a day for up to two weeks out of every month.

Keep your iron up. Try to consume more iron from herbs and food sources on the days that you bleed heavily, says Susun. You'll feel more energetic and alive within two weeks, and your flooding will diminish noticeably by your next period, she adds.

Herbal sources of iron include dandelion leaves, milk thistle seed, Angelica sinensis, black cohosh, echinacea and peppermint, according to Susun. Food sources of iron include leafy greens, tofu, raisins and sultanas, carrots, beets, pumpkin, tomatoes, cauliflower, mushrooms, soya beans and salmon. Of course, lean red meat is the best source of iron because it contains haeme iron, which is more readily absorbed by the body than iron from vegetable sources.

Reach for yellow dock root. Another iron source, yellow dock root contributes one milligram of iron per 20-drop dose of alcohol tincture or per three-teaspoon dose of vinegar tincture, says Susun. Yellow dock also contains thiamine and vitamin C, which assist absorption of iron, as well as compounds, called anthraquinone glycosides, that stimulate bile production, thereby aiding digestion and nudging a sluggish liver. Either an alcohol or a vinegar tincture is fine, taken daily in tea or water, she advises. Iron is absorbed a little at a time, so she suggests taking it throughout the day.

Limit 'iron-eating' foods. Coffee, black tea, egg yolks, bran and supplements containing more than 250 milligrams of calcium impair iron absorption, Susun notes. Limit consumption of coffee and tea, and take your calcium at night or with meals that don't include iron-rich foods.

LOW LIBIDO

If hitting an unexpected speed bump with your car equates to the best sex you've had lately, you know your hormones are sending you a signal.

Nearly three out of four women suffer from some kind of sexual difficulty, whether it's decreased sex drive, vaginal dryness or trouble reaching orgasm. Even if we don't have any severe sexual dysfunction, nearly all of us, according to one survey, have at least one sexual concern.

In the past, the best advice doctors usually offered to improve our sex lives – if we had the courage to ask – ran from drinking a glass of wine to buying some lingerie. Most commonly, they'd claim it was all in our heads.

And it's true that emotions and relationship issues are indeed a huge part of desire and sex. But researchers are discovering that quite often the problem lies in our hormones, which become more erratic as we age.

But getting older doesn't have to equate with making love less often. In one study, women over the age of 65 had almost 10 per cent more sex than women aged 39 to 50. Drug companies, inspired by men's reaction to the arousal drug Viagra, are discovering an equally enthusiastic, untapped market in women.

SIGNS AND SYMPTOMS

LOW LIBIDO

Plummeting oestrogen levels during menopause can lead to minimized sensation in the labia, interfere with lubrication, and make the tissues in the vagina very delicate and prone to bleeding. In one study, 67 per cent of menopausal women experienced low arousal and pain during sex, and 92 per cent reported trouble reaching orgasm.

The good news is that the enormous amounts of research resulting from this quest provide numerous ways we can preserve our sexual function *without drugs* and knowledge we can use now to have better sex *tonight*.

What Can You Do?

For women who find themselves less interested in sex at menopause, experts suggest:

Recall pleasurable sensual experiences. Of course, good sex begins long before you even set foot in the bedroom. 'Reconnecting to powerful feelings of sensuality – not necessarily sexuality – can go a long way towards helping you feel desire,' explains Dr Gina Ogden, a leading sex therapist.

'Sometimes these playful, sensual memories predate adult sexual experience – like the time you went skinny-dipping when you were eight years old. Summoning the energy that infused your joy as a little girl can revitalize your sex life today,' she says.

Stay physically active. Regular exercise will relieve stress, improve your mood, and help you feel great about your body, says Dr Yula Ponticas, a clinical psychologist in the Sexual Behaviors Consultation Unit at Johns Hopkins University School of Medicine.

When researchers looked at women aged 50 and older, they found that those with the highest levels of physical fitness were also the ones who enjoyed intimacy more often.

Aerobic exercise wakes up your nerves and primes your sympathetic nervous system for sex, says Dr Cindy Meston, a professor of psychology and sex researcher. It also improves your cardiovascular system and increases blood flow, a key part of arousal and orgasm.

Yoga, a more sedate exercise, may also help, says Dr Deborah Moskowitz, a naturopathic doctor.

Get your blood flowing. Stimulating herbs that get blood circulation flowing enhance sexual feelings in women, notes Aviva Romm, a herbalist. 'With more blood flow to the pelvis, you'll feel more aroused.'

Simmer these herbs in 480 ml (16 fl oz) of water for 20 minutes: 1 tablespoon of grated fresh ginger, 7 to 10 cloves, 2 or 3 cinnamon sticks, 4 or 5 black peppercorns and 7 to 10 cardamom pods. Strain and add small amounts of milk and honey to taste. If you wish, add ¼ teaspoon of vanilla. 'Vanilla comes from the orchid family, and orchids are incredibly sensual flowers,' says Aviva. 'It's an aphrodisiac.'

Use the right lubricant. Vaginal dryness is a prime cause of painful intercourse, so you may be tempted to reach for the petroleum jelly – but that's not a good idea. Petroleum jelly can break down condoms. Plus, it isn't water-soluble, so it remains in the vagina, where it can harbour yeast and other infection-producing microbes.

So what's the better option? Try vaginal lubricants such as Astroglide and KY jelly, which are designed to relieve friction during sex by coating your vaginal walls. Unlike moisturizers, they tend to evaporate and often need to be reapplied during intercourse. For more tips on overcoming vaginal dryness, turn to page 158.

If you smoke, quit. Women who smoke complain of vaginal dryness and painful intercourse a lot more than non-smokers do. The reason? Smoking restricts the blood flow necessary for a clitoral erection, engorgement of the vaginal walls and labia and lubrication.

Consider hormonal help. If the strategies above don't help, you may want to consider testosterone therapy. Several studies have shown that supplementary testosterone (in tablet or injection form) can increase sexual arousal in some postmenopausal women, especially in women whose ovaries have been removed.

Your doctor can explain the benefits and drawbacks of testosterone therapy.

Medical Alert

LOW LIBIDO

Ask your doctor to refer you to a gynaecologist if your sexual desire continues to wane despite having tried measures such as those described in this chapter. You may have an underlying health problem, such as chronic fatigue syndrome, depression, Lyme disease or a thyroid disorder. And if you suspect that an emotional conflict is sapping your sexual desire, consider getting counselling from a psychotherapist or sex therapist. See Chapter 6 for some ideas on rekindling your sexual fire.

MEMORY PROBLEMS

You walk into the living room to get something – but what? You drive right past the supermarket and forget to turn in. What's going on?

The connection between memory and menopause has long been an issue of debate. In ongoing research into brain function, scientists are trying to determine whether oestrogen receptors or oestrogen metabolites (the breakdown products of oestrogen) affect memory function. But so far nothing has been proved, says Dr Adelaide Nardone, a gynaecologist.

In recent research at Yale University, magnetic resonance imaging (MRI) was used to study the influence of oestrogen on the brain patterns of postmenopausal women. Therapeutic doses of oestrogen affected brain activity in memory tasks, like remembering a just-looked-up telephone number. This seems to support the theory that oestrogen aids short-term information storage.

This small study provides a tantalizing clue to oestrogen's role in brain function, but definitive links have not been forged, says Dr Nardone, who believes that much of menopausal 'mental misfiring' can be traced to fatigue.

Women undergoing the change of life are prone to insomnia and night sweats, which often leave them exhausted, she says. And increased anxiety about memory lapses may further distort their perception of memory loss.

What Can You Do?

If you want to remember better naturally, work these easy remedies into your daily routine. The first two tips are helpful if your memory problems are sleep-related. The others will help to boost your memory power any time of day.

Practise good 'sleep hygiene'. Be sure that your bedroom is dark and shielded from noise so you can sleep beyond 6 am. Eliminate any stimulating input, she says – no watching TV in bed. Take care not to eat any heavy foods after 7 pm as vigorous digestion tends to inhibit deep sleep. The same goes for caffeine and chocolate, which can keep you awake.

Take a sip of milk. If restorative rest still eludes you, Dr Nardone suggests taking 300 to 500 milligrams of calcium (a glass or two of fat-free milk will do the trick) an hour before bedtime to encourage sleepiness. Calcium may soothe the body into a deep sleep that is interrupted less often, she says.

Get some mental exercise. The more you challenge your brain, the better it'll perform. Any kind of mental exercise, such as doing crossword puzzles, can help improve your memory. Just be sure it's something you enjoy; if you don't enjoy the activity, it won't feel as rewarding.

Get physical. In one study, researchers found that volunteers who took an hour of aerobic exercise three times a week performed better on memory tests than those who didn't work out. Exercise, they speculate, may increase oxygen flow to the brain and speed glucose metabolism, improving recall. Exercise can also reduce stress, which can interfere with memory.

SIGNS AND SYMPTOMS
MEMORY PROBLEMS

For many women, menopause and forgetfulness seem to arrive hand in hand. Frequent memory lapses, sudden blanks and forgotten names can be frightening and may lead you to believe that you're not as sharp as you used to be.

Medical Alert

MEMORY PROBLEMS

If your memory seems to be failing steadily, don't hesitate to consult your doctor. Many treatable conditions can cause forgetfulness – among them, depression, drug side-effects and thyroid disorders. Your doctor can determine whether or not you have age-related memory impairment or something more serious.

Make meaningful connections. To remember things like street addresses or a shopping list, make up a story or a sentence that links that information in a meaningful way. To remember someone's address – for example, 65 South Street – tell yourself, 'Sixty-five is my retirement age, and many people move to the South of Europe after they retire.'

Paint a mental image. Concrete visual images can help connect new names. Assume that you meet a prospective boss, Ms Saucer, at a job interview, and her most striking feature is her green eyes. Picture saucers painted to look like huge green eyes. So, later in the conversation, or the next time you meet her, her eyes will remind you that her last name is Saucer.

Avoid distractions. Make a mental note of what you're going to do before you do it. It will minimize distraction, which makes you forget why, for example, you walked into the living room. You head for a room to find something in particular, but as you enter, something else catches your attention.

So, instead, tell yourself, 'I'm going into the living room to get the photo album,' for example, and you will be less likely to get distracted by the magazines and papers on the coffee table.

NIGHT SWEATS

It's one thing to feel a hot flush spread from your chest to your neck and your head, leaving you sweaty and flushed during the day. Hot flushes are uncomfortable, inconvenient, and sometimes embarrassing, but after your first few hot flushes, you realize, as other women approaching menopause do, that you can deal with them.

Nocturnal flushes – night sweats – are a different story. Waking up in a pool of perspiration disrupts your sleep. So does getting up from a deep sleep to change your soaking wet nightclothes and sheets.

'But night sweats, hot flushes and the chills that sometimes follow are nothing to worry about and last only nine to 16 months, on average,' says Dr Lila A. Wallis, a professor of medicine. It's believed that the drop in the production of the female hormone oestrogen and other hormonal changes interfere with the way the body regulates heat.

Nightly heat waves may be harmless and temporary, but that's no consolation if you can't get the rest you need.

In addition, some experts believe that some of the mental symptoms attributed to hormonal changes before and after menopause – foggy thinking, for instance – are more likely a result of sleep deprivation.

What Can You Do?

If your sleep time suddenly becomes hot and steamy for all the wrong reasons, try these simple strategies to help you sleep through your next night sweat (or get back to dreamland in a wink).

Have a cup of sage tea before bed. Sage – an ordinary kitchen herb – can help reduce or sometimes even eliminate night sweats, according to herbalists. To make a sage infusion, place four heaped tablespoons of dried sage in a mugful of hot water. Cover tightly and steep for four hours or more. Then strain, reheat and drink. (Used in therapeutic

SIGNS AND SYMPTOMS

NIGHT SWEATS

Night sweats are hot flushes that occur during sleep. You wake drenched in sweat, sometimes several times a night. Because night sweats disturb sleep, you're often tired during the day.

> *Medical Alert*
>
> # NIGHT SWEATS
>
> If you haven't slept well in weeks and generally feel under the weather, make an appointment with your doctor, who can give you even more advice on eliminating night sweats.

amounts, sage can increase sedative side-effects of drugs. Do not use medicinal amounts of sage if you're hypoglycaemic or undergoing anticonvulsant therapy.)

Sleep on all-cotton sheets and pillowcases. Cotton is a breathable fabric that draws moisture away from the skin. Avoid cotton/polyester blends, nylon and satin – they'll leave you feeling hot and clammy. And keep a light cotton quilt at the foot of your bed to pull over yourself if you get the chills after a hot flush.

Wear cotton. Wear all-cotton underwear and short-sleeved, knee-length nightgowns (long-sleeved gowns will be too hot and uncomfortable). Avoid nylon or polyester blends, which will trap rather than release heat. Keep a dry nightie handy at the foot of your bed or on a chair next to your bed. If you have to change in the middle of the night, you won't have to get out of bed and rummage through your drawers.

Keep the right supplies on hand. Leave a small cotton towel next to your bed to wipe the sweat off your chest, neck and face, and place a fan next to your bed to cool those heat waves.

Drift back to sleep. Try keeping your eyes closed and letting yourself drift into that semi-conscious state between sleep and waking. You will be more likely to fall back asleep, says Dr Sonia Ancoli-Israel, a professor of psychiatry.

Get out of bed. If you can't fall back to sleep within 15 to 30 minutes, get out of bed and do something relaxing for half an hour, such as reading. Then try to go back to bed. Repeat as often as you need to until you fall asleep.

PAINFUL URINATION

To some extent, women get urinary tract infections (UTIs) simply because of their anatomy. Because the rectum, vagina and urethra are within centimetres of one another, it's easy for infection-causing bacteria such as *Escherichia coli* to enter the urinary tract. And at menopause, normal changes in the vaginal tissues can contribute to UTIs. Most women will experience at least one or two UTIs at some time in their lives.

If the infection is limited to the urethra, it's called urethritis. More often than not, the infection travels further up the tract and into the bladder and becomes cystitis (or, simply, a bladder infection). Treatment usually consists of a one-day or three-day dose of antibiotics. Unless treated promptly, a bladder infection can move to the kidneys, leading to a more serious condition, called pyelonephritis.

Anything that alters the bacterial balance of the genito-urinary tract can render women more susceptible to UTIs.

Women who use certain birth control methods – for example, spermicides containing nonoxynol-9 – are at higher risk for UTIs. This ingredient is found in spermicidal jellies, spermicidal foams or inserts and condoms with spermicidal lubricant.

What Can You Do?

While UTIs require a doctor's care, you can ease the pain and protect yourself from future infections with this expert advice.

Drink more water, not less. You may be tempted to drink less because urinating afterwards is so painful. But if you drink a few litres of

---

SIGNS AND SYMPTOMS

PAINFUL URINATION

Painful urination is often a sign of a urinary tract infection (UTI). Other symptoms you may experience are a burning sensation when urinating, frequent urination, voiding just a few drops at a time and passing blood.

Medical Alert

PAINFUL URINATION

If you have more than two UTIs (or what you think are UTIs) in six months, or more than three episodes in 12 months, see a doctor and get a urine sample for an accurate diagnosis. Also, see your doctor if your UTI symptoms are accompanied by blood in the urine, chills, nausea, vomiting or lower-back pain.

If you've received a prescription for your UTI and symptoms don't start clearing up within two days, call your doctor promptly.

---

water within 24 hours of discovering UTI symptoms, you might be able to flush the bacteria out of your system.

Fix a bicarbonate of soda cocktail. At the first sign of symptoms, mix ½ teaspoon of bicarbonate of soda in a 240-ml (8-fl oz) glass of water and drink it. The bicarbonate of soda raises the pH (acid–alkaline balance) of irritating, acidic urine.

Get juiced. Cranberries contain unique substances called condensed tannins that make it more difficult for bacteria to adhere to the lining of your urinary tract. Accordingly, drinking cranberry juice can both prevent and treat UTIs. In several published studies, drinking just three 240-ml (8-fl oz) glasses of cranberry juice a day significantly reduced the incidence of UTIs in elderly women.

Doctors caution, however, that in some women with urinary tract sensitivity, cranberry juice may act as an irritant because of its high acid content. If cranberry juice seems to make your symptoms worse, try diluting it before stopping it altogether.

Wear stockings or pop socks and skirts or loose trousers. If you have an infection, wearing tight undergarments or jeans forces the bacteria that normally line your vaginal area up into your urethra. If you have irritation, constrictive clothing can worsen pain and discomfort because it presses against the already inflamed urethral opening.

Cut other offenders. Whether you have a simple irritation or an infected urinary tract, the last thing that you need are known bladder irritants. The most notorious bladder irritants are citrus fruit, tomatoes, mature cheeses, chocolate, spicy foods, caffeine, alcohol and nicotine. For certain people, anything carbonated – especially beer and soft drinks – may irritate the bladder and make you urinate more frequently or urgently.

Ask about oestrogen cream. If you suddenly start experiencing more UTIs as you approach menopause, you may want to ask your doctor about oestrogen cream. Applied topically, it helps your body maintain a normal vaginal environment and helps the urethra to produce mucus; both of these protect against bacterial infections such as UTIs.

SNORING

So, you think you don't snore? Think again. Ever wake up with head-aches? Morning fatigue? In women, these symptoms can be signs of sleep apnoea, interruptions in sleep when you actually stop breathing several times a night. This disorder affects the quality of your sleep, making you restless during the night and tired during the day.

'Snoring is a key sign of sleep apnoea in men and women alike, but women are less likely to know they snore,' says Dr Joan Shaver, one of the first researchers to study sleep problems in women. 'If a man snores, his wife will complain and prompt him to find a solution. But if a woman snores, often the guy won't notice because he's too busy snoring himself.'

But there may be other factors at work as well. When women suddenly start snoring, for example, it's usually a sign that oestrogen is plummeting. As this hormone drops, it affects the sensory nerves in the soft palate, causing it to lose muscle tone and become flaccid. As you sleep, the soft palate flaps, creating the lovely sound known as snoring.

SIGNS AND SYMPTOMS

SNORING

Snoring can be a symptom of sleep apnoea, a breathing disturbance char-acterized by explosively loud snoring interspersed with pauses of silence. During those pauses, which can last ten seconds or longer, the snorer actually stops breathing. Because these episodes typically happen dozens of times each night, the snorer awakens feeling unrefreshed and exhausted.

Medical Alert

SNORING

Apnoea is a serious disease that may increase your risk of stroke, high blood pressure or an enlarged heart. And the longer it goes undetected, the worse it can become because apnoea worsens with age. So see your doctor for a complete evaluation if snoring doesn't respond to self-care after a few weeks.

Menopausal weight gain, also known as the Buddha belly, is another culprit. As belly fat crowds the internal organs, pushing them up and putting pressure on the diaphragm, you have to work harder to breathe. Forcing the air in and out causes you to snore. Hypothyroidism can also be the reason that some women snore. A sluggish thyroid aggravates sinus problems; plus, it contributes to weight gain. Menopause itself triggers hypothyroidism in many women; about 60 per cent of all Western women have an underactive thyroid by the age of 70.

What Can You Do?

Short of buying your partner earplugs, give these tips a try. If you don't see improvement in a couple of weeks, see your doctor to rule out a more serious underlying condition.

Change sleeping positions. Snoring is usually worse when you sleep on your back, so try elevating your head, which may reduce soft palate flapping. Sleeping on your side is another good option for many.

Use a decongestant. Low-dose, over-the-counter decongestants may help keep your sinuses open during the night. Take the smallest dose you can, as decongestants can keep some people awake.

Take your oestrogen by moonlight. If you're on oestrogen replacement therapy, take it at night. This will enhance sleep, too, guiding you to a deeper level faster.

Kick the butts. Smoke may cause swelling and inflammation of the throat tissues which, when swollen, are more likely to vibrate and produce snoring. Add this to your list of 1,001 reasons why it's a good idea to give up smoking.

Drop that drink. Alcohol relaxes all the muscles in the throat that vibrate. And it's dose-related – the more you drink, the louder you'll snore.

UNWANTED FACIAL HAIR

In up to 90 per cent of women with unwanted facial hair, there is no underlying problem. But for the other 10 per cent, such problems could be caused by a tumour, polycystic ovary syndrome or a benign condition called hirsutism, in which hair grows fast and thick on the cheeks, chin, forehead and chest.

Oral contraceptives, hormone replacement therapy and a prescription drug called spironolactone (which reduces the amount of male hormones floating around in our bodies) may help remove unwanted facial hair.

What Can You Do?

Of course, you can always follow the tried and tested: shaving, waxing, depilatories and electrolysis. Here's what the experts have to say about each method.

Ready, set, shave. Shaving is by far the easiest way to remove unwanted hair; try a double-edged razor for the closest shave. And contrary to the old wives' tales, shaving facial hair doesn't cause it to grow back faster or coarser.

Pick up a waxing kit. Waxing pulls hairs out by the roots, which can be painful depending on your tolerance. It's best for light, fuzzy hairs you'd rather live without. As far as the waxing options are concerned, most

---

SIGNS AND SYMPTOMS

UNWANTED FACIAL HAIR

As we age and our oestrogen levels drop, problems with unwanted facial hair may worsen. If this scenario applies to you, you're not alone. About 25 per cent of normal middle-aged women have unwanted facial hair.

> **Medical Alert**
>
> # UNWANTED FACIAL HAIR
>
> If you experience any sudden change in hair growth – especially in those areas where men typically sprout hair, such as the cheeks – see a doctor to rule out an underlying health condition.

women find that the prewaxed plastic strips aren't as painful to use as warm wax that hardens as it cools.

With sugaring, a variation of waxing, hair is coated with a paste of sugar and wax – it's easier to pull off than wax and therefore less traumatizing to the skin.

Take the chemical route. Chemical depilatories are creams that contain chemicals to dissolve hair, so they're best for places on the body where the skin is not easily irritated. To ensure best results before using a depilatory for the first time, smear a little on 2.5 cm (1 in) of your forearm, let it sit for the amount of time specified on the packaging, and then wipe it off. Wait 24 hours before proceeding so that you can see if symptoms such as itching, redness or irritation develop.

One advantage to depilatories is that some contain hair growth inhibitors and fruit enzymes – ingredients that interfere with the protein that lets hair grow back.

Make an appointment for a permanent solution. Electrolysis is the only permanent hair removal option. But you can't do it yourself – a professional performs it in a beauty salon or a specialist hair removal centre by inserting a probe into each individual hair follicle and passing an electric current through it. Removing all of the hair on your upper lip may require several sessions.

Make sure that you choose a highly experienced technician since improper electrolysis can leave permanent scars.

WEIGHT GAIN

Even medical experts can't agree whether it's ageing or menopause that causes extra weight to migrate towards the middle. They just know that the average Western woman puts on up to 7 kg (15 lb) during late adulthood, most of it around her waist. One reason is that ageing causes your metabolism to slow down and your lean muscle mass to decrease. Since lean muscle cells burn more calories than fat, the less muscle you have, the fewer calories you burn. Add to this the fact that the shape of your body is determined by muscle strength, and it's no surprise that as muscles grow weaker, paunches start.

Now think back to puberty and childbirth, two other major hormonal shifts in your life. Both events triggered changes in body composition and weight. Menopause is no different, except that as your oestrogen decreases, a subsequent increase in insulin makes losing weight more difficult.

Even women who don't gain weight can see 4.5 to 7 kg (10 to 15 lb) shift to the waist, an effect of ageing known as central obesity. Osteoporosis magnifies the problem as it causes the spine to shrink, shortening the waistline.

Besides making you feel unattractive, extra weight around your middle is sometimes associated with cardiovascular disease, high blood pressure and an increased risk of breast cancer. What's the best way to combat abdominal spread? Sensible eating and exercise.

Don't deprive yourself of too many calories, or your body will go into starvation mode, which lowers your metabolism even more. Try to follow a

---

SIGNS AND SYMPTOMS

WEIGHT GAIN

If you're even 20 per cent overweight — say you should weigh 54 kg (8½ st) but tip the scales at 65 kg (10 st 4 lb) — your health risks soar for high blood pressure and cholesterol, diabetes and other diseases. Luckily, the news is not all bad. Dropping even 4.5 kg (10 lb) excess weight can significantly lower your cholesterol and your blood pressure.

low-fat diet and do some kind of aerobic exercise for at least 30 minutes three times a week to boost your metabolism and burn fat. Weight-bearing exercise, such as walking, will also strengthen your bones and help to prevent osteoporosis.

And don't look to hormone replacement therapy (HRT) as some kind of magic answer. Research to date is inconclusive. One study found that women on HRT gained more weight than those not on HRT, while another study found that HRT appeared to prevent the increase in abdominal fat. Any decision regarding this type of therapy should be based on your overall health, not on your desire to lose weight.

As you move through menopause, try not to curse your fat cells. They help convert other chemicals in your body into oestrogen, which may ease your transition by reducing the incidence and severity of hot flushes, mood swings and sleep disturbances.

What Can You Do?

If ever there is a time in your life to accept yourself, menopause is it. Concentrate on being fit and healthy rather than squeezing into the jeans you wore when you were first married. The following advice may help.

Keep a food diary. Write down not only what you eat but also how much you eat, when you eat it, and what you're doing at the time. This process helps you shape healthier dietary habits by uncovering hidden sources of calories and fat. It also identifies situations that switch on your appetite – for example, you may realize that you consistently turn to food when you are bored or stressed-out.

Trim 600 calories a day from your present diet. The simplest way to do this is to eat less. You can also switch from whole milk to skimmed or semi-skimmed, order foods such as fish and potatoes baked instead of fried, switch to reduced-fat mayonnaise and salad dressing, and take similar small calorie-saving steps.

Eat half as much. Do you usually fill your plate or, if you're eating at a restaurant, eat everything that you're served? Instead, try eating half as much. Chances are, you'll be able to meet your nutritional needs without feeling deprived.

Increase your physical activity level. Find little opportunities to be more active throughout the day, and you'll give yourself a huge boost towards reaching your weight-loss goals. If you walk to work, for example, tack an extra couple of streets onto your route. You'll burn 10 more calories per day, or roughly 3,500 more calories per year – the number of calories in about half a kilo (one pound) of fat. Some other strategies are to take the stairs instead of the lift, go for a brisk walk at lunchtime, and park your car at the far end of the car park when you go to the supermarket.

Create the changes that count. For best results, some experts recommend that you make only one or two minor changes at a time in your eating and exercise habits. For example, look for ways that you can cut your calorie intake by roughly 125 calories a day. You might try putting mustard instead of mayonnaise on your sandwich or using skimmed instead of full-fat milk in your coffee or tea. Same goes for exercise. Start with a ten-minute work-out and gradually build from there. By going slowly and giving yourself time to adjust to the lifestyle changes you make, you set yourself up for lasting weight loss.

Make a date with the weight. If you use scales to monitor your progress, weigh yourself at the same time every day. Your weight fluctuates over the course of 24 hours. Stepping on the scales in the morning one day and at bedtime the next can leave you with an inaccurate (and discouraging) picture of how you are doing.

MAKING THE MOST OF YOUR MEDICAL OPTIONS

Modern women have the option to do many things that our grandmothers never dreamed of – ride whitewater rapids, work shoulder to shoulder with men, and postpone or entirely bypass child-bearing. Unlike women of a century ago, whose average life expectancy was 47 years, women today can expect to live at least 30 years beyond menopause. And while the very term *postmenopausal* fills many women with anxiety, even dread, we all would probably agree that it certainly beats the alternative.

Of course, in order to make the most of those extra years, you'll want to continue in the best possible health. And that means staying informed about the latest health issues and getting the care you need before small problems become serious. This chapter will discuss some of the issues you may encounter as you make your way through the world of conventional medicine. Are there any good reasons to take hormone replacement therapy? Does breast cancer risk decrease – or increase – after menopause? When the doctor suggests a hysterectomy, do any other options exist?

What can you expect when facing a disease? But first, read on for advice on working with your doctor.

Make the Most of Your Doctor Visits

If there's one fact about medical care that doctors and patients whole-heartedly agree on, it's that there isn't enough time in the average visit to cover everything. In fact, research shows that most doctors are so pressed for time that they tend to interrupt a patient, on average, after 23 seconds.

With that in mind, here's how you can beat the time crunch and get the most from every visit.

Be up-front and early. When you make an appointment, briefly tell the receptionist what your issues are. She can help determine how much time you need with the doctor. And to avoid a long wait when you arrive, try to get the first appointment of the day. Or call just before your appointment to find out if the doctor is behind schedule.

Discuss the biggest issues first. Prepare a list of key points that you want to bring up and, during your visit, start with the most important ones.

Present your complaints chronologically. For instance, if your first symptom of dizziness started two months ago, then got worse a month ago, then became a constant problem last week, say so. If you lost your balance and fell in the past two days, this type of background information should help your doctor put things in perspective.

Explain your strategy. Let your doctor know what, if anything, you've done to try to remedy your condition. Tell her if you've changed your diet in any way or taken any vitamins, herbs or over-the-counter remedies. Describe their effects, if any, on your symptoms.

Say yes to tests. Your doctor may suggest different tests, depending on your age, medical history and current symptoms. If you pay for private medical care, you can request these yourself; otherwise, they will be undertaken at your doctor's recommendation. They might include:

- Mammogram, to spot early signs of breast cancer.
- Pelvic examination, along with a manual breast check and digital rectal check.

- Blood pressure screening. High blood pressure (indicated by readings consistently above 140/90) is a risk factor for heart disease and stroke.

- Cholesterol screening. These tests measure your total cholesterol, LDL, HDL and triglycerides.

- Complete head-to-toe skin examination by a knowledgeable physician to detect any signs of skin cancer.

- Serum oestradiol test to help gauge the onset of menopause.

- An electrocardiogram (ECG). More than one-third of the women who have heart attacks don't have any warning signals beforehand. An ECG can help spot heart damage that you may not be aware of.

- A thyroid function test, which involves lab analysis of a blood sample.

- Faecal occult blood test to reveal any hidden blood in your stool, which can be a warning sign of colon cancer and other diseases.

- Bone density screening to help determine your risk of developing osteoporosis. In many cases, women only need this test once.

MAKING THE HORMONE DECISION

Scared and confused about whether or not to take hormone replacement therapy (HRT)? You're not alone.

'The doctors are confused, so I can't imagine that women aren't,' says Dr Machelle M. Seibel, a clinical professor of gynaecology and obstetrics and a reproductive endocrinologist.

So what's causing all the confusion? In case you missed the big news, 16,000 participants in the Women's Health Initiative (WHI), a landmark study of hormone replacement therapy, opened their post to find a letter that said, 'Stop taking your tablets.' The researchers sent the letter after they'd found a higher risk of breast cancer among users of a combination HRT (a mixture of oestrogen and progestogen), plus increased risks for heart attack, stroke and blood clots.

To make matters more frightening, the FDA in the US recently used these findings to declare *all* forms of oestrogen to be known carcinogens. This stance has been taken up by cancer research organizations world-wide.

Now, thanks to these alarming headlines, many menopausal and post-menopausal women don't know *what* to think about hormone replacement therapy. And with so many millions of us heading into menopause, plus greater numbers to come, a lot of us are left scratching our heads.

So, should you take HRT or not? When you read through all the research, it essentially boils down to this: HRT is not the source of all women's evils as its critics say, but neither is it the cure-all that others claim.

Basically, you're facing an individual decision as unique as you are. Along with your doctor, you need to consider your health, family medical history, risks and your own gut feelings, says Dr Sharon Youcha, a gynaecologist with a special interest in menopause.

Making Sense of the Headlines

What troubles most of us isn't what we know about hormone replacement therapy – it's what we don't know, or at least don't know enough about. The real risk of breast cancer in conjunction with HRT is still up in the air. Meanwhile, one of the potential benefits of long-term HRT – prevention of heart disease – has been called into question. Here's what we know for sure.

The Breast Cancer Connection

Ask any woman considering HRT about her greatest concern, and she'll probably tell you: breast cancer. The spectre of this dreaded disease looms large over our decision regarding hormones. In fact, some experts say that it's the number one reason holding most women back.

But in evaluating your individual risks, it's important to recognize that

THE MILLION WOMEN STUDY

Results from the Million Women Study, a UK research project investigating reproductive and lifestyle factors affecting women's health, has found that women who use or have used hormone replacement therapy (HRT) are more likely to develop breast cancer, compared to women who have never used HRT. This is the largest study to date linking the menopausal treatment to an increased breast cancer risk. Researchers noted that the risk of breast cancer was higher among women who used combined oestrogen/progestogen forms of HRT, rather than oestrogen alone.

Led by Valerie Beral of the Cancer Research UK Epidemiology Unit in Oxford, the study reviewed medical data from over one million women aged 50 to 64 who enrolled in the study between 1996 and 2001. Approximately 50 per cent of the women were using or had used HRT. Key findings included the following:

* Postmenopausal women who used combined oestrogen/progestogen methods of HRT were twice as likely to develop breast cancer, compared to women who never used HRT.
* Women who used oestrogen alone were 30 per cent more likely to develop breast cancer and women who used tibolone (a steroid that combines oestrogen, progesterone and androgene activity, comparable to standard HRT) were 45 per cent more likely to develop breast cancer, compared to women who never used HRT.
* The increased risk of breast cancer appeared to decrease after a few years off treatment.

Based on these findings, the charity Cancer Research UK estimates that for every 1,000 postmenopausal women who use HRT for 10 years, beginning at age 50, there will be five additional cases of breast cancer among women using oestrogen alone and 19 additional cases among women using oestrogen/progestogen combination regimes. Overall, Cancer Research UK estimates that HRT contributed to an additional 20,000 cases of breast cancer during the past decade, 15,000 of which resulted from combined oestrogen/progestogen HRT.

Experts have welcomed the results of the study, but have pointed out that HRT may still be appropriate for women with a low risk of breast cancer and severe menopausal symptoms, for a short period of time. In a previous publication, the authors themselves have urged people to be cautious in interpreting the findings from this study. This is because the design of the study is weaker than the US WHI trial so the conclusions are not as reliable.

both truth and exaggeration exist in the information that's presented to us. The key is to put it all in perspective. And the first step is to understand the links between hormone replacement therapy and breast cancer.

A cancer cell forms when the DNA that controls cell division is damaged. By stimulating breast cells to divide, oestrogen increases the chance that one of those new cells will have damaged DNA and will then multiply out of control, causing cancer.

Studies show that women who take HRT for five years or less – the usual amount of time required to treat menopausal symptoms – probably have little to worry about, except for a very small risk of blood clots.

Questions arise for women who take HRT for longer. More than 50 population studies found that the risk of breast cancer increased approximately 30 per cent for women who used HRT for five years or more. And it's possible that progesterone – added to oestrogen replacement therapy to reduce the risk of endometrial cancer – actually *increases* the risk of breast cancer. In the landmark WHI study, which was suspended after five years, researchers saw a 26 per cent increase in the number of breast cancer cases among HRT users.

But before you flush your Premarin down the toilet, consider what those numbers actually mean, a reality that is often lost in the hysterical headlines. According to the authors of the WHI study, for every 10,000 women taking hormone replacement therapy, 38 cases of invasive breast cancer would occur, eight more cases than you would expect to see in a group of women not taking HRT. So taking HRT long-term may increase your *personal* risk of developing breast cancer, but probably only slightly.

Future research seeks to clarify the link between HRT and breast cancer. Until then, you and your doctor have to make decisions based on your history and, obviously, your comfort level. If you're lying awake at night worrying about breast cancer, then you shouldn't be taking HRT.

Hormone Replacement Therapy and Heart Disease

For years, many doctors viewed HRT as the ultimate line of defence against osteoporosis and heart disease – two problems that plague women most after menopause.

Years of observational studies backed up this theory by showing that women who took the hormones had fewer heart attacks than those who didn't. Other studies found that women on HRT saw their LDL ('bad') cholesterol levels drop by about 10 per cent, while their beneficial HDL cholesterol increased by about 9 per cent.

But a four-year study of 2,700 women in the US, part of the Heart and Estrogen/Progestin Replacement Study (HERS), found in 1998 that women who already had heart disease were 50 per cent more likely to have a heart attack during their first two years on HRT than those not taking hormones. The WHI backed up these results, revealing that compared with the group not taking HRT, 22 per cent more participants developed cardiovascular disease while taking HRT.

HOW DO THEY MAKE PREMARIN?

The safety and effectiveness of oestrogen aren't the only controversies swirling around hormone replacement therapy. How some forms of oestrogen are made has people up in arms as well.

The oestrogen that many doctors prescribe today is called conjugated equine oestrogen, better known in prescription form as Premarin, one of the most prescribed drugs in the country. The word 'equine' gives you a hint – Premarin is derived from the urine of pregnant mares. Mares produce high levels of oestrogen in their urine until the middle of their third trimester.

The controversy comes on two fronts. On one side, animal rights activists believe that breeding horses just so the mares can produce oestrogen-rich urine is cruel. They also claim that the foals of these pregnant horses are unwanted 'by-products'.

On the other side are those who feel women shouldn't put a substance such as horse urine into their bodies and that they should be using 'natural', or bioidentical, oestrogens processed from plants.

'Some women view the oestrogen in Premarin as an unacceptable choice because it is derived from pregnant mares. But for the majority of women I see, it is a point of interest but not a point of decision making. Would they rather it came from a plant or some other source? Yes. But I don't think that alone is going to stop women from taking oestrogen,' says Dr Machelle M. Seibel, clinical professor of gynaecology and obstetrics and a reproductive endocrinologist.

The bottom line is that if you have heart disease and are considering HRT for osteoporosis or perimenopausal symptoms, you should find other treatment options. If you haven't had a heart attack and don't have severe arteriosclerosis, you're probably fine taking HRT for short-term relief of menopausal symptoms.

But heart disease prevention shouldn't be the reason you're taking HRT, anyway. The cholesterol benefits you get from hormones are about the same as you'd get from a low-fat diet. And cholesterol-lowering statins and other medications provide better protection.

The Good and the Bad

Think of the decision to take HRT as a set of scales: you weigh the benefits on one side, the drawbacks on the other. Whichever side tips the scales determines your decision. But before you start weighing, you have to know the facts.

The Pros

Bones. Next to calcium, oestrogen is probably the biggest ally we have in the quest for strong bones. Basically, it increases factors that stimulate bone to grow. So when we lose oestrogen in middle age, we begin losing bone.

If you take HRT, studies show that bone loss slows. One study found that women who took HRT for five or more years reduced their risk of back and neck fractures by 50 to 80 per cent. Another series of studies found that women taking hormones reduced their risk of hip fractures by 25 per cent. Once you go off HRT, however, you're likely to lose whatever gains you've made.

Hot flushes. Without question, hormone replacement therapy is the most effective treatment for hot flushes and other perimenopausal symptoms, says Dr Deborah Kwolek, an expert in women's health. Women who take HRT reduce their hot flushes by up to 70 per cent.

For many women, Dr Youcha adds, HRT is the only way to get through menopause without investing in a towel company. How does it help? One theory is that as oestrogen declines during menopause, a chemical called luteinizing hormone (LH) rises, possibly throwing off the way your body's thermostat works. HRT affects the release of that hormone, stabilizing the thermostat.

Sleep. Oestrogen helps you get a better night's sleep. A study conducted in Turku, Finland, found that HRT eliminated the hot flushes, night sweats and headaches that kept women up at night. Another study, at Brown University Medical School in the US, found that in menopausal women, HRT helped alleviate sleep apnoea (in which you stop breathing several times during the night). Somehow, researchers speculate, oestrogen helps stimulate breathing during sleep.

Mood. It could be the result of getting a better night's sleep, or it could be that HRT actually helps regulate mood, but women on hormone replacement therapy often report feeling less irritable, says Dr Wulf H. Utian, executive director of the North American Menopause Society.

Memory. The studies aren't completely conclusive yet, but research suggests that oestrogen replacement therapy helps improve memory and cognitive function and may even ward off or at least slow the progression of Alzheimer's disease.

Weight. In what may be the greatest incentive to take HRT, researchers at Boston University discovered that women on hormone replacement therapy had significantly less body fat than non-HRT users. And a study at Johns Hopkins University found that HRT increased muscle mass while decreasing body fat. Researchers speculate that it's the oestrogen drop that contributes to the all-too-common postmenopausal weight gain.

The Cons

Blood clots. Hormone replacement therapy more than doubles your risk of developing blood clots in your legs, which could dislodge and travel to your lungs (causing a pulmonary embolism) or to your brain (caus-ing a stroke or other serious problems). Oral oestrogen elevates blood-clotting factors produced by the liver, which may trigger the formation of blood clots.

Gallstones. HRT also slightly increases your risk of developing gallstones. Oestrogen stimulates the liver to remove cholesterol from the blood

and divert it into the gallbladder, and gallstones form if too much cholesterol flows into the gallbladder.

Endometrial cancer. Because the additional oestrogen stimulates the
cells lining your uterus to continue to divide, using oestrogen therapy
alone can increase your risk of this cancer. But that risk is essentially eliminated when progesterone is added to the hormone mix.

Periods. Just when you thought it was safe to throw out the tampons,
you start on HRT and begin having periodic vaginal bleeding again.
Blame HRT. This is the main reason women stop taking hormones.

Side-effects. Like most drugs, HRT has a long list of possible side-
effects, including severe stomach pain or swelling, pain or numbness in the
chest, shortness of breath, severe headaches, changes in vision and breast
lumps. Other, less serious side-effects include bloating, breast pain and tenderness, nausea, headaches and mood swings.

Restrictions. You may not be able to take hormone replacement
therapy if you've had breast cancer, liver disease, large uterine fibroids or
endometriosis because HRT may aggravate these conditions.

Questions to Ask Yourself

Now it's time to put all the pros and cons on the scales. How do you
weigh it out? Try answering these few simple questions, Dr Utian suggests.
Along with your doctor's input and recommendations, your answers will
help guide you down the right path.

'Do I have perimenopausal symptoms such as hot flushes?' If
the answer is no, you don't need HRT.

'Why do I need hormone replacement therapy?' You should not
take hormones just because you're a menopausal woman. Your doctor
should clearly state why she thinks you need HRT and what your long-
term plan of action should be.

'What does my medical history show?' You'll have to go over this
with your doctor, but many women either underestimate or overestimate
their own risks of certain diseases. You may fear breast cancer, but your
family history and your own bone density may predispose you much,
much more to osteoporosis.

'**Are there other options?**' Obviously, lifestyle changes can make a big difference. And there are other drugs on the market that help treat hot flushes and bone loss. That's not necessarily to say these are better than HRT. In fact, you may find that hormone replacement therapy is perfect for you. But look at all your other options before deciding.

'**How do I feel about HRT?**' Gut feelings go a long way, Dr Youcha says. If taking HRT 'seems right' medically, but you're anxious about it, talk to your doctor about the alternatives.

Customizing Your HRT Plan

'Gone are the days of one-size-fits-all hormone replacement therapy, when all menopausal women received a standard dose of oestrogen and progestogen and either lived with the results or abandoned the therapy altogether,' says Dr Andrew M. Kaunitz, professor of obstetrics and gynaecology at the University of Florida Health Science Center and director of gynaecology and menopause services at the University of Florida Medicus Diagnostic Center. Today hormone replacement therapy uses various forms of oestrogens (such as conjugated oestrogen, oestradiol or esterified oestrogen) and progestogen (such as medroxy-progesterone acetate or micronized progesterone) in various doses. 'If you stopped taking HRT – or are worried about starting – because of side-effects like headaches or spotting, don't assume it's not for you. Unpleasant side-effects can be reduced or, in most cases, eliminated,' says Dr Kaunitz.

To find the hormone mix that's best for you, talk to your doctor about tailoring therapy to your needs. Here are your options.

Continuous combined. Oestrogen is taken along with a low dose of progestogen every day. The constant dosage of progestogen (which signals the uterus to shed its lining) means that you may experience erratic bleeding or spotting, with no pattern or regularity. For some women, this eventually stops.

Sequential/cyclical. Oestrogen is taken every day and progestogen is taken on a cyclical schedule so that bleeding occurs on a regular, predictable schedule, as if you're having a period.

Quarterly progestogen. Another option is to take oestrogen every day and progestogen every three months, or quarterly throughout the year. You'll have just four periods per year.

Low-dose oestrogen. Taken in a very low dose with no progestogen, oestrogen produces none of progestogen's PMS-like symptoms, and the dosage of oestrogen is low enough that there appears to be no increased risk of endometrial cancer. Your doctor, however, may recommend regular tests of the endometrium if you choose this option.

Pill, Patch or Cream?

The form in which you take hormone replacement therapy can be as important as the type and dosage that you take. The most common method of administering HRT is orally, either with separate tablets for each hormone or with a combined pill.

HRT is also available in a patch, which is ideal for women who find taking tablets unpleasant, who have problems absorbing the oral medication, or who have high triglyceride levels.

Hormone cream, applied topically inside the vagina where it has an immediate effect, works especially well for women who experience sexual discomfort after menopause and tolerate neither tablets nor the patch. Topical treatments have such a low dose that progestogen may not be necessary, but they don't treat hot flushes or protect your bones the way a tablet or patch does.

Interested in natural hormone replacement therapy? See page 248.

WHAT YOU NEED TO KNOW ABOUT BREAST CANCER

With all the races, the pink ribbons and the celebrities talking about their breast cancer, it's difficult to ignore the disease. And we shouldn't ignore all the hype because close to 35,000 UK women get breast cancer each year. In Australia over 7,500 women are diagnosed with the disease each year and in New Zealand some 2,000 new cases are diagnosed. The International Agency for Research on Cancer (IARC) estimates that there are 1.2 million new cases of breast cancer each year and 500,000 deaths from breast cancer worldwide.

Although oestrogen is considered a key player in breast cancer – in both its advent and its progress – there are two schools of thought on how much of a role it actually plays.

THE INVENTORS OF HORMONE REPLACEMENT THERAPY

Maybe we're the first generation openly talking about taking hormones for health, but we aren't the first ones who thought about it. There's evidence that more than 5,000 years ago, Chinese emperors ingested the urine of young women to gain the restorative powers of hormones.

In the modern era, we can thank the research team of Edgar Allen and Edward A. Doisy. They got the ball rolling on the hormone revolution in 1923 with their landmark paper in the *Journal of the American Medical Association*, 'An Ovarian Hormone: Preliminary Report on Its Localization, Extraction, and Partial Purification and Action in Test Animals.'

The two met in their medical school library in the early 1920s and quickly became friends. So when Dr Allen wanted to make extracts from ovarian tissue, because of previous research that showed removing the ovaries from rats stopped their oestrus cycle (basically, an animal's menstrual cycle), he asked his good friend Dr Doisy to help. The two set about identifying the hormone that turned out to be oestrogen.

As for the progesterone part, they got some help from G. W. Corner and Willard Allen, who identified and explained the role of progesterone in 1927. Then in 1929, Dr Doisy – continuing his previous oestrogen research – actually crystallized oestrogen, which was originally called theelin. So by the end of the 1920s, scientists understood and could re-create the roles of both oestrogen and progesterone in a woman's body.

Ironically, Dr Edgar Allen was just 31 and Dr Doisy only 29 when they published the findings that would later change the science of ageing.

Some research suggests oestrogen may do to our breast cells what too many desserts do to our fat cells – make them grow and divide. And if any of the breast cells are already cancerous, oestrogen feeds their growth. The other school disagrees and sees oestrogen as more protective than causative in breast cancer development. If you do develop breast cancer while on oestrogen, it will typically be a type that is more easily treated.

Unfortunately, passing the menopause milestone doesn't seem to lower your chances of oestrogen–positive breast cancer.

The older you get, the greater your chances of getting breast cancer. One reason may be that although your ovaries no longer make oestrogen after menopause, there's still enough oestrogen hanging around in your tissues to stimulate breast cancer cells to grow.

Yet despite the theories and recent headlines, steering clear of oestrogen replacement therapy won't completely remove your breast cancer risk. 'In fact, most breast cancer cases occur in women who are postmenopausal and have never been on hormone replacement therapy,' says Dr M. Michelle Blackwood, a breast surgeon.

Another theory suggests that we get more breast cancer as we age because of the overall deterioration our bodies undergo, not the oestrogen. 'We're at the highest risk of breast cancer when we have the *least* oestrogen in our bodies,' says Dr Blackwood.

Progesterone, too, causes cells in the breasts to divide, says Dr Malcolm Pike, a professor of preventive medicine. A study conducted at screening centres throughout the United States and published in the *Journal of the American Medical Association* looked at 46,355 postmenopausal women who had used hormone replacement therapy (HRT) in the previous four years and found that the breast cancer risk of women who had taken oestrogen alone increased by 1 per cent each year they took the therapy. The risk of women who had taken an oestrogen/progesterone combination increased by *8 per cent* each year they continued that therapy.

Testosterone may also play a part. Women with breast cancer have 30 to 100 per cent more testosterone than healthy women do. It's not known exactly what testosterone does in breast tissue to increase the risk. One theory suggests that it stimulates breast cells to grow and

REDUCE YOUR BREAST CANCER RISK

Worried about breast cancer? You can start reducing your overall risk today with a number of small lifestyle changes.

Fill up on colourful foods. Want to lower your risk of cancer? Then eat at least seven servings of fruit and vegetables in all hues of the rainbow every day. That's because carotenoids, the plant chemicals that create bright colours in fruit and vegetables, may help prevent cancer. So make it a habit to dine on blueberries, grapes, raisins, plums, dark green lettuce, spinach, kale, carrots, strawberries, tomatoes, beets and red, green, orange and yellow peppers.

Try a new fruit or vegetable each week and learn new ways to prepare old favourites. You don't have to give up meat completely; just shift towards a more colourful, plant-based diet. A good tool for expanding your produce menu is a vegetarian cookbook.

Slim down. More fat equals more unopposed oestrogen (oestrogen without a progesterone parent keeping it under control), which increases your risk of breast cancer. So a lean body means less oestrogen and a lower risk of breast cancer.

Take your breasts for a walk. A study conducted at the Keck School of Medicine of the University of Southern California showed that women who had exercised at least four hours per week for at least 12 years and hadn't gained much weight in adulthood were 29 per cent less likely to get breast cancer than women who had never exercised at that level.

Make it a virgin cocktail. Your arteries may feel pretty good after a few drinks, but your breasts have a low tolerance. A combined report of more than 50 studies found that drinking as few as two alcoholic drinks a day can increase your breast cancer risk by 25 per cent, no matter whether you drink cheap vodka or a fine red wine.

divide, increasing the odds that one of those cells will have the cancer switch turned to 'on'.

Hormones also play a role once the cancer has developed. Some breast cancers have receptors for oestrogen or progesterone, sometimes referred to as ER-positive and PR-positive. On the one hand, it's good to have a hormone-sensitive tumour, because it's more likely to respond to hormone-blocking drugs such as tamoxifen (Nolvadex). On the other

SHE FOUND A LUMP

At 48, Helene Kosakowski felt very tired. Then one day she found a lump in her breast. It turned out to be oestrogen-sensitive breast cancer.

'I never did routine checks on my breasts,' says Helene. 'I was a nurse, and I taught other women to do them, but I never performed them on myself. I didn't think it could happen to me.

'When I did find a lump, I went straight to my doctor. He sent me for a mammogram immediately.

'When they repeated the mammogram a few times, I knew something was wrong. Being a nurse, I wasn't about to leave without talking to the radiologist, so I was able to look at my film that day. The lump looked like a small sphere. It had fingerlike protrusions, so I knew it had spread. I was given an appointment with a surgeon for the following week, and I left for a family holiday.

'Needless to say, I was panicked throughout the week-long break. I still had some hope that it wasn't cancer. When I returned, the surgeon put my hope to rest – it was cancer. And from the biopsy, he could tell that the tumour was oestrogen-sensitive, meaning the cancer cells were using oestrogen to grow. He scheduled my surgery – a lumpectomy (removal of the tumour) and a partial mastectomy (removal of part of my breast) – for 7 March, which was my birthday.

'Then, in April, I had a modified radical mastectomy (removal of my entire breast) and an axillary dissection (removal of some of my lymph nodes) because

hand, ER- or PR-positive breast cancer is fuelled by oestrogen or progesterone, so you have to be extra careful to avoid exposure to those hormones.

Understanding Tamoxifen

Tamoxifen is a great treatment for the majority of breast cancers, especially oestrogen-sensitive ones. But doctors are hesitant to prescribe the drug to *prevent* breast cancer, mainly because it can increase the risk of endometrial cancer. So before you decide to take tamoxifen as a preventive measure, you should carefully examine the pros and cons.

It might be worth it to take tamoxifen if you're genetically at risk for breast cancer. Then your risk of getting breast cancer is higher than your risk of getting endometrial cancer from the drug. If you still have your

the cancer had spread. I chose not to have breast reconstruction. Instead, I wear a prosthesis.

'Six months of chemotherapy followed. Emotionally, this was a terrifying time. Every day, I just got up and tried to make things as normal as possible. I drove myself to chemo. It was still business as usual. If I went on social outings or travelled with my husband, I simply put on a scarf and a hat and dressed myself up.

'After my chemotherapy was complete, I started taking tamoxifen (Nolvadex). Tamoxifen stops oestrogen from being produced in my body so the hormone won't feed the cancer. Tamoxifen has its downsides; it brings on hot flushes, weight gain and the fear of endometrial cancer. My treatment ended 18 months ago, and since then I've been able to lose weight and start exercising again.

'Today, aged 54, I'm doing well. I devote a lot of my time to voluntary work for a cancer charity, helping women who are going through the same thing I did. And this past year, I travelled to the capital to share my experience with MPs to press cancer bills and issues.

'If I can give any advice to women going through a bout of breast cancer, it's that you have choices. You don't have to have a breast reconstruction. I never had one. I look good and have a nice body, except I'm missing a breast and wear a prosthesis. It's your body, and you need to look at all the choices before you make a decision.'

uterus, doctors will carefully monitor you with ultrasound for any signs of endometrial cancer and any endometrial thickening. They should do occasional biopsies to look for any tissue changes. If you've had a hysterectomy, you don't have to worry at all about endometrial cancer.

Obesity seems to worsen the effects of tamoxifen on the endometrium. In postmenopausal women, a reaction can occur in body fat that actually creates the most potent form of oestrogen – oestradiol – which can feed endometrial cancer cells. So if you're overweight, you should give tamoxifen careful thought and talk to your doctor about your options.

Another catalyst for endometrial cancer is oestrogen replacement therapy. If you're on this, you're already at an increased risk for endometrial cancer. In that case, the tamoxifen may be the straw that breaks the camel's back. Make sure you discuss this with your doctor.

Stay in Touch with Your Breasts

Unless the Queen invites you to lunch on the day you are due to have a mammogram, keep your appointment. And frankly, there's no excuse for not making a monthly breast self-examination part of your regular health routine. 'Early detection can really make a difference in the long-term outcome,' says Dr Donna Sweet, a professor of internal medicine. Roughly 90 per cent of the time, breast lumps are found through self-examination.

So regardless of whether you've gone through menopause or not, the importance of these tests simply cannot be emphasized enough. (See 'Why You Still Need Mammograms' on page 309.) Experts recommend that all women perform a monthly self-examination and women over the age of 50 should have a mammogram every three years. If you have a mother or sister with breast cancer, get one every year from 35 onwards.

Try to do your self-examination at the same time every month, ideally five to seven days after your period ends. Begin by standing in front of a mirror with your hands at your sides. Raise your hands and hold them together behind your head. Look for any change in the size or shape of your breasts, as well as for nipple discharge, redness, puckering and dimpling. Next, press your hands on your hips, pull your shoulders and elbows forward, and look for similar changes.

After this visual examination, you need to check your breasts again by touch. Follow a definite pattern, and make sure that you repeat it the same way every time – it's the best way to ensure you'll notice anything out of the ordinary. Three common examples that experts recommend are the circle, the wedge and the vertical patterns.

To use the circle pattern, your fingers travel in small circles, moving from the outer portions of your breast towards the nipple. With the vertical pattern, you slide your hand up and down in vertical lines from one side of the breast to the other. Similarly, with the wedge pattern you start from the nipple and work your fingers out to the edge of your breast and then back towards the nipple again.

Whatever pattern you choose, make sure that you cover one breast thoroughly before proceeding to the other one.

Visualize a Pain-free Mammogram

In order to examine as much of the breast as possible during a mammogram, the breast is compressed between an x-ray plate and a plastic cover. For many women, this image alone is enough to make the prospect of a mammogram unnerving – not to mention fear of a cancer diagnosis.

'Just about every woman experiences a certain degree of apprehension when getting a mammogram,' says Dr Laurie Nadel, a doctor of clinical hypnotherapy who has coached many women in calming mammogram nerves. Her own first mammogram was so painful that she put off scheduling another one for years. 'I used mental imagery to pick up the phone and make another appointment.' The trick is to give yourself a boost by remembering a positive experience, she adds.

If your mammogram appointment is just around the corner, practise this exercise three times a day, then again just before you step up to the mammography plate. Ball up your hands into fists. Close your eyes and think about a wonderful place where you once felt calm, relaxed and safe. Remember the sights, sounds and smells as you relive every moment.

To enhance your sense of peace, add more colour to that picture-perfect place in your mind. Make the images larger or sharper, or increase the tightness of your fists, until your calmness reaches its peak.

As your anxiety slowly fades, release your hands, shake them out and open your eyes. To recapture that warm, fuzzy feeling, make those fists again and say to yourself, 'Take me back.'

The more you practise this exercise, the faster your brain will make the connection between your fists and total calm, says Dr Nadel. 'The painful part takes three seconds, then it's over. If you learn to quickly flood your body with feelings of happiness, you'll reduce the perception of anticipated pain.'

To further reduce discomfort, try to schedule your mammogram about a week after the last day of your menstrual period, when breast swelling and tenderness are minimal. This may not be possible, but it's worth asking. And a few weeks before your appointment, cut down on caffeine and start taking 200 to 400 IU of vitamin E daily.

HOW TO AVOID
SURGERY-INDUCED MENOPAUSE

If you're one of the thousands of women a year who are told by their doctors, 'You need a hysterectomy,' don't panic. Maybe you need surgery, and maybe you don't.

Each year, more than 70,000 women in the UK undergo hysterectomies (removal of the uterus) for fibroids, endometriosis and abnormal bleeding. That's a figure that is, head for head, reflected around the West; for example, in Australia 30,000 hysterectomies are performed each year. If a woman's ovaries are also removed, her oestrogen levels plummet, and she is thrown full-tilt into menopause. And even if the ovaries are preserved, there's some evidence that menopause will occur earlier as a result of a hysterectomy. Overall, it's the second-most-common surgery in the West among women in their reproductive years. (For those who've gone through natural menopause, it's far less frequent.)

There's some startling news. About 90 per cent of women who had the surgery could have been offered uterus-sparing treatments instead, says Dr Brian Walsh, a gynaecological surgeon. That's important if you still want to have children or want to avoid an early menopause.

So why aren't we told about other options? 'Doctors are either unaware of the alternatives or just not comfortable with performing the procedures that require higher levels of skill,' says Dr Mitchell Rein, an obstetrician-gynaecologist, reproductive endocrinologist and associate professor at Harvard Medical School. Hysterectomy should be necessary only if a woman's condition doesn't improve after she has explored all other possibilities, or if she has invasive uterine cancer, says Dr Rein.

Cancer accounts for fewer than 5 per cent of all hysterectomies, says Dr Walsh. Non-life-threatening conditions make up the rest.

Following are three of the most common conditions that normally prompt a hysterectomy and the ways to treat them that don't involve removing your uterus. If your doctor doesn't mention any of these options, ask, especially if you still want to have children.

Fibroids

As many as four out of ten hysterectomies are done to remove fibroids, or uterine leiomyomas, bundles of muscle and connective tissue that can grow inside or outside the uterus. Uterus-saving treatments include:

Ibuprofen. Over-the-counter pain relievers like ibuprofen (such as Nurofen) can sometimes help ease the pain and heavy bleeding of fibroids. For mild symptoms, they should be your doctor's first line of treatment, says Dr Rein.

Uterine artery embolization. This non-surgical procedure cuts off the blood supply to the fibroid, causing it to shrink, says Dr Linda D. Bradley, director of hysteroscopic services in the department of obstetrics and gynaecology at the Cleveland Clinic Foundation.

Recovery is quick, and side-effects are few, but the impact on fertility is questionable. 'After a woman has this procedure, we don't know if her uterus is strong enough to sustain a pregnancy,' says Dr Bradley.

Myomectomy. This surgical technique removes fibroids but leaves the uterus intact. The size of the fibroids and where they occur determine what type of myomectomy your doctor performs. With a hysteroscopic myomectomy, fibroids are removed vaginally. In laparoscopic surgery, the doctor extracts fibroids through a small incision made in the abdomen. The more complex procedures for multiple and large fibroids are done through larger abdominal incisions, says Dr Rein.

For more information about the new hope for fibroids, turn to page 304.

Endometriosis

About one out of five hysterectomies is done for endometriosis, where fragments of the uterine lining grow outside the uterus in the abdomen and on the ovaries. Fuelled by oestrogen, the tissue then grows and bleeds on a monthly cycle, causing chronic pain, inflammation, scar tissue and other problems. Fortunately, because of the oestrogen connection, this is one condition that usually slows the closer you get to menopause. Other ways to control endometriosis include:

Oral contraceptives (birth control pills). Most effective for milder cases of endometriosis, oral contraceptives alter the balance of oestrogen and progesterone, slowing the progression of the disease, says Dr Walsh.

Hormonal drugs. GnRH agonists are powerful hormonal drugs that reduce oestrogen production and shrink endometrial tissue. The most commonly used are Leuprorelin (Prostap), Goserelin (Zoladex), Nafarelin (Synarel), Buserelin (Suprecur) and Triptorelin (Decapeptyl). However, there are two problems with these drugs. First, they send you into early – but reversible – menopause. Second, they can cause premature bone loss if used long-term, says Dr Rein.

Laparoscopic surgery. With this surgery, possibly performed when endometriosis is diagnosed, stray endometrial tissue is destroyed with an electrical device or a laser, says Dr Walsh. Endometriosis has a tendency to recur, but birth control pills can help keep it in check.

Laparotomy. More invasive than laparoscopic surgery but less so than hysterectomy, this procedure destroys the endometriosis tissue and/or associated scar tissue.

Abnormal Bleeding

Persistent or heavy bleeding accounts for another 20 per cent of hysterectomies performed. Other options to consider:

Ibuprofen. In mild cases, NSAIDs such as Nurofen can sometimes help slow down the bleeding, says Dr Walsh.

Hormone treatment. Contraceptives like Depo-Provera, administered by injection, or regular birth control pills are often ideal for women who are not ovulating regularly and who are bleeding throughout the month, says Dr Walsh.

Endometrial ablation. This destroys the lining of the uterus and the layer under it, and the procedure can be done vaginally. Ablation will usually leave you infertile. And while one-third of all patients will have no more bleeding, one-third will have spotting or a light flow. Twenty-five per cent will have average periods. A few – 5 to 10 per cent – will be no better off than before.

FACING DISEASE

'The stinging shock of cold water…'

'An unexpected slap in the face…'

'Hearing voices in the room fade as the sound of your pounding heart fills your ears…'

Every woman has different words to describe her first moments after receiving an unexpected diagnosis. And while the reactions may differ, the flood of questions that follow are usually similar. What's next? What should I expect? What are my options?

That's why we've put together this guide to facing the conditions most common to women as they approach menopause. After all, knowledge is power. And if you know the basics of what to expect, you're already a step ahead.

Breast Cancer

If you detect a lump or if anything else seems abnormal during your monthly self-examination, see your doctor. Your doctor will check your breasts in at least two positions, such as lying down with your arms raised over your head and then standing or sitting upright. This will help your doctor get a complete sense of the size, shape and texture of any suspicious lumps.

Then, if your doctor suspects anything abnormal in your breast, she may refer you to a specialist for further tests such as a mammogram or an ultrasonogram, which uses high-frequency sound waves to determine if a lump

DON'T GO IT ALONE

When it comes to facing disease, two heads are definitely better than one. If you're undergoing treatment for a serious health condition, consider asking a relative or close friend to go to your medical appointments with you. Talk beforehand about the questions you have so that your companion knows what information you need to get from your doctor.

is solid or fluid. If those tests confirm her suspicions, then a biopsy is usually the next step. This can be done with a special needle, or the surgeon may opt to cut out all or part of the lump. Once the lump is removed, a pathologist will examine it to look for cancer cells.

If cancer is confirmed, treatment will depend on several factors, including the size of your tumour and whether it has spread to the lymph nodes or other parts of your body. You will likely receive a combination of surgery, radiation and/or chemotherapy. Surgery for breast cancer used to mean one thing: mastectomy. A lumpectomy, which removes only the tumour, followed by radiation is far more common now, however.

Radiation therapy uses very sophisticated equipment to direct high-energy rays at cancerous tissue, thereby killing cancer cells in their tracks. Another variation of radiation therapy involves placing radioactive implants into your breast. In some cases, both forms of treatment are warranted. Typical side-effects may be limited to a sunburn-like burn on the treated breast, fatigue and the loss of underarm hair near the treated breast.

Chemotherapy, which may involve a variety of anti-cancer drugs, is a standard treatment for premenopausal women whose breast tumours are greater than one centimetre in diameter. Because these drugs travel through the bloodstream, they are often able to destroy cancer cells that other treatments may miss. This treatment is more frightening for many women because of its reputation for nasty side-effects, including hair loss, nausea, vomiting and loss of appetite. But in many cases, these side-effects can be controlled or eliminated.

Heart Disease

Heart disease takes many forms, from heart attack to stroke to chronic chest pain, and involves just as many methods to diagnose it. For example, your doctor may begin a physical examination with a blood pressure reading. Blood tests may also be ordered as cholesterol problems help advance heart disease.

From there, you could be referred for further tests depending on your risk factors, health history and symptoms. These may include an electrocardiogram, a chest x-ray, an exercise stress test or a nuclear imaging test. A non-invasive test known as electron beam computed tomography (EBCT) rapidly scans the beating heart with x-rays to examine any potential problems in the arteries. This test is so effective that it can detect heart disease in women who have no outward symptoms.

Depending on your diagnosis, your doctor may prescribe preventive medicines. These commonly include a class of drugs called statins, which reduce cholesterol and consequently lower the risk of having a first heart attack. Low-dose aspirin therapy has also been shown to prevent recurrence of heart attacks among women who've already had them. Long-acting beta-blockers are usually prescribed for chronic chest pain.

If a blockage is detected, there are several surgical procedures that doctors use to restore proper blood flow through the heart. With balloon angioplasty, a doctor inserts a catheter, or tube, into a narrowed artery and inflates the balloon. This allows him to implant a wire-mesh tube within the walls of the artery to keep it from closing again. Bypass surgery is another option, and in this arena there's good news especially for women – there's now a less invasive type of bypass surgery, in which the incision is made under a breast instead of down the middle of the chest. Of course, it's not an appropriate approach for all cases, but it's definitely worth discussing with your doctor if you need bypass surgery.

Mood Disorders

If you perceive your moods to be especially volatile as you move through menopause, share your concerns with your doctor. You may find that getting an accurate diagnosis can be the first step towards feeling better. For many, it's a relief to be able to put a name and label on what they are experiencing.

As far as treatment is concerned, there are many antidepressant drugs available to help correct chemical imbalances in the brain. Your doctor should ask a lot of questions about your symptoms and general health to determine which drug treatment would be best for you. In most cases, it may be several weeks before you notice its effect.

About 60 to 70 per cent of people who can tolerate the side-effects of antidepressants get better with the first drug they take. If after eight to 12 weeks you feel that the particular prescription isn't working for you, talk to your doctor about trying another antidepressant.

In part, your medical history will determine how long you need to take these drugs. Previous episodes of depression usually indicate that a longer time frame is in order.

Women who combine talk therapy with prescription medicines often do better in the long run. Two short-term and highly effective methods to consider are cognitive behaviour therapy and interpersonal therapy.

In a cognitive behaviour session, your therapist will help you focus on changing behaviour and improving mood by identifying which situations make you happy and which lead you to feel depressed. You'll then examine your behaviour and thought patterns and find ways to change them. Interpersonal therapy, on the other hand, focuses on your personal and social interactions with others and how they affect your mood. Basically, you'll work on improving your relationships so that you feel better about yourself.

Osteoporosis

If you are at or beyond menopause, have experienced a fracture, or have one or more risk factors for osteoporosis, experts strongly recommend that you have the appropriate medical tests to determine your bone mineral density. Knowing your bone density is really the only way to detect the disease before a fracture occurs or to predict your chances of another break, as well as to monitor the rate of bone loss.

Presently, the best test for determining your bone mineral density is called DEXA (dual-energy x-ray absorptiometry). Don't let the name unnerve you – the test is painless, non-invasive and brief (usually about 10 to 20 minutes). With very low dose radiation, the DEXA machine will scan your hips and spine, two areas where osteoporosis can have the gravest consequences, and compare your bone density with that of the average woman. A reading between -1 and -2.5 standard deviations from normal indicates low bone mass. A standard deviation of $+1$ or $+2$ is great news, showing you have good bone density.

If you've been diagnosed with osteoporosis, you should repeat this test every two years to make sure that your treatment is working. If your initial score was very low – more than 2.5 standard deviations below normal – talk to your doctor about having it rechecked annually.

As far as treatment is concerned, osteoporosis is a unique disease in that it doesn't 'belong' to a particular medical speciality. Most likely, you would be referred to a gynaecologist first; however, there are three other types of experts who may be called upon as needed: an endocrinologist, who treats hormone-related conditions; a rheumatologist, who specializes in diseases of the joints and connective tissues; or an orthopaedist, who deals with skeletal problems.

There are also some new drugs available to prevent and treat osteoporosis. One of the most recent contenders, teriparatide, takes a new approach in treating osteoporosis because it helps restore the body's ability to build new bone, rather than slowing bone loss. Other drugs include raloxifene (Evista), which is a selective oestrogen receptor modulator (SERM) drug that imitates oestrogen without the same potentially harmful effects, such as raising the risk of breast cancer. Raloxifene has been shown to increase bone mass in the spine and hips and to reduce the risk of fractures in the spine by up to 50 per cent. Other drugs making a difference include alendronate (Fosamax), which is especially effective for reducing spine and hip fractures, and a companion drug called etidronate (Didronel PMO). Risendronate sodium is another bisphosphonate drug used only in women after the menopause. Calcitonin, a hormone that slows bone loss and modestly builds spinal bone density, is a common treatment for women at least five years beyond menopause. Calcitriol is a vitamin D-like compound that can be used in osteoporosis following the menopause or in situations where osteoporosis is caused by steroid drugs.

Reproductive Cancer

Endometrial cancer can occur before or after menopause; but since the number one symptom is abnormal bleeding, it's easy to detect, fortunately. For this reason, any bleeding after menopause, even simple spotting, warrants a trip to the doctor right away. Ovarian cancer, on the other hand, is more difficult to diagnose because its symptoms mimic everyday female complaints – cramping, bloating and swelling in the abdomen. What's more, a family history of ovarian cancer is the biggest risk factor for the disease, so there aren't a lot of hands-on things you can do to reduce your risk. Any symptoms that persist for longer than a month should be evaluated by your doctor.

Most endometrial cancer is caught fairly early and treated with a hysterectomy. More advanced cases may require removing the ovaries, fallopian tubes, nearby lymph nodes and upper part of the vagina. Sometimes follow-up includes radiation treatments, hormone replacement therapy or chemotherapy.

The primary treatment for ovarian cancer is surgical removal of the tumour. If the case is more severe, one or both ovaries, nearby organs and lymph nodes may be removed as well. Unfortunately, because surgery rarely cures ovarian cancer, chemotherapy is usually prescribed.

Chapter

9

THE WIDE WORLD
OF ALTERNATIVE
TREATMENTS

IF YOU'VE BEEN WATCHING THE NEWS, YOU'VE PROBABLY HEARD plenty about alternative treatments for the menopause. With the sudden fall in the number of women using conventional hormone replacement therapy, our news media are filled with headlines about the latest options. Ironically, much of this 'late-breaking news' comes from healing traditions that are thousands of years old! But what you might not have heard about natural healing is that alternative medicine offers a lot of satisfaction beyond healing. Because many alternative treatments help integrate the healing of mind and body and put *you* in control of your treatment options, they can also help restore vital balance, perspective and meaning to life in the menopausal years. This chapter is a guide to alternative options. You'll learn about natural plant-based hormone alternatives as well as the wide range of supplements you can pick up at your healthfood shop. Plus, we'll cover all of the other great healing methods, such as acupuncture and yoga, used by women around the world to treat menopausal symptoms. But first, let's talk about what you should do before you make any changes that could affect your long-term health.

Coordinate Your Care

If you decide to add a herb or supplement to your diet, or if you're interested in trying out an alternative therapy, tell your doctor about your plans. She may need to monitor your progress or adjust your medication. In some cases, a herb or supplement may have a dangerous interaction with a drug you're already taking (see 'Using Herbs and Supplements Safely' on page 331). And be patient. Don't expect natural healing methods to work in quite the same way that Western medicine does. 'We're used to quick-fix treatments that work almost immediately,' says Dr Adrian Fugh-Berman, former head of field investigations for the Office of Alternative Medicine at the National Institutes of Health in the US. 'Natural medicine tends to be slower, gentler, and often easier on your system.' So listen to your body, find what works for you and give it time.

TRAVELLING DOWN A DIFFERENT ROAD: HRT ALTERNATIVES

For some women, the answer to the hormone replacement therapy (HRT) question is a clear no. Whether it's because you can't take HRT – or you just won't – there are plenty of other options that can help you deal with the symptoms of perimenopause and safeguard your health.

Natural Hormone Therapies

If you are interested in hormone replacement therapy but concerned about the side-effects, you might want to try 'natural' hormones that are derived from plant compounds and are identical to the progesterone and oestrogen your body produces. Though plant-derived hormones have actually been in use for a long time, the natural hormone therapies, when compared with conventional HRT, offer similar relief from symptoms without the number or severity of commonly reported side-effects, such as depression, breast tenderness and bloating.

Bear in mind, however, that another point of contrast concerns the research. Hands down, there have been many more studies conducted to determine the effects (and risks) of conventional hormone replacement therapy – but natural hormone proponents are quick to point out that you simply can't take conclusions drawn from the studies of conventional HRT and apply them to the use of natural hormones. They are quite different medicines. To explain more, here's an overview of your options and what we know about how natural hormones can help.

Why Do I Need Hormones Again?

Your body is designed to produce just the right amounts of oestrogen and progesterone to keep the rhythm of your menstrual cycle balanced and regular throughout your reproductive years. Oestrogen is the hormone that revs up at the beginning of each cycle and makes sure that ovulation occurs every month. And then progesterone steps in to help regulate your cycle and nourish the lining of your uterus in preparation for pregnancy, should this occur. But its job is also to prevent oestrogen from causing the lining to thicken too much. So when an egg is not fertilized, progesterone levels drop, causing the lining to be shed in a menstrual period. This is important because it is the monthly shedding that helps lower the risk of endometrial cancer.

As you approach menopause, your ovaries slow down and stop pro- ducing progesterone, and you ovulate less frequently or not at all. By the time you reach menopause, the drop in progesterone is almost 100 per cent. Oestrogen, in contrast, drops by about 90 per cent since there are other sources of oestrogen in the body.

Decreased oestrogen levels are to blame for virtually all menopausal symptoms. So if you're given oestrogen to counter them, you're also typ- ically prescribed a progestogen (the synthetic version of progesterone) to prevent the oestrogen from causing a build-up of tissue in your uterus that can lead to cancer.

Though a progestogen acts like your body's own progesterone in its ability to counter the potentially cancer-causing effects of oestrogen, your body may well be able to tell the difference. Progestogens appear to be the culprit behind many of the unpleasant side-effects that some women experience with HRT. By comparison, side-effects are rarely reported among those using natural progesterone, which is derived from wild yams, soya beans and other plant sources.

But Do Natural Hormones Really Work?

Unfortunately, there have been few scientific studies on natural progesterone. In fact, scientists know little about the progesterone you make in your body, let alone the kind made in a lab. But we do know that natural progesterone – which, despite its name, is also created in a lab – is chemically identical to the hormone secreted during the luteal phase of your menstrual cycle, which is the two weeks after you ovulate.

The reason you need a lab to intervene is that wild yams and soya beans do not contain progesterone but rather another chemical – a plant compound called diosgenin – that can be turned into a facsimile of your own progesterone, but only in a lab. Until recently, natural progesterone was too quickly absorbed to do the body any good. That's another important difference between synthetic and natural – progestogens are easily absorbed.

If you hate tablets and are wondering about the natural progesterone creams, it's true that progesterone in this form is more readily absorbed through your skin. Studies have found, however, that it's difficult for a woman to achieve normal levels of circulating hormone by applying it to the skin.

As far as oestrogen is concerned, when a woman chooses natural hormone replacement therapy as an alternative to conventional treatment, she uses different combinations of either two or three types of oestrogen (identical to the two or three oestrogens that her body makes on its own). The working names for these combinations are biestrogen and triestrogen. The exact combinations and the oestrogens used to mix them are prescription items prepared by a compounding pharmacist – that is, they are mixed in much the same way that old-fashioned pharmacists once formulated medications, so you get the individualized dosage ordered by your doctor. (If you can't locate a compounding pharmacist or chemist in your area, your doctor can direct you to one.

Herbs

If your menopausal symptoms are limited to a few unpleasant problems that you'd rather do without, perhaps a herbal product can help. But there are so many different herbs. A knowledgeable herbalist, for example, may draw on thousands of different healing plants, and your average healthfood shop or chemist may stock dozens upon dozens of herbal products. Which ones do you need? To answer just that question, we've compiled detailed profiles of the ten safe, easy-to-find herbs that top British and American practitioners consider to be among the best choices for problems that concern women the most in the years before and after menopause. So they're a great place to begin your journey into the ancient and nurturing world of botanical home remedies.

In this section, you'll also learn what makes each herb valuable and unique. Each profile highlights useful information about the herb as well as the botanical name and other common names. Knowing a plant's Latin name is important to help ensure that you gather or purchase the right herbal remedy because it's the name by which it will be known no matter where you are. A herb's common name can vary from region to region or from country to country, making it difficult to be sure what you're using.

You'll also discover how people throughout history – from the ancient Greeks to Native Americans, from Europeans of the Renaissance to early-twentieth-century practitioners – used each herb, tracing the link between ancient healing arts and the ways women use herbal remedies today. Most importantly, you'll learn the specifics of what's available and how different types of herbs and herbal products can help you.

Use these handy profiles to get acquainted with herbs before you explore their use. And refer to them often to refamiliarize yourself with the herbs' potential benefits. Safe use guidelines begin on page 331.

Agnus Castus (Vitex)

Botanical Name: *Vitex agnus-castus*

To understand the history of agnus castus, it may help to know that its Latin name means pure, innocent or chaste – not surprisingly, in ancient Athens women used it to quell sexual passion and sacrificed it to the goddess Ceres as a symbol of chastity. The medieval herbalist Gerard called agnus castus the perfect herb for celibates. In nineteenth-century France, vitex syrup was given to 'suppress the desires of Venus'. It's little wonder, then, that some of the other names for agnus castus include chasteberry and monk's pepper.

Modern herbalists don't subscribe to the notion that agnus castus dampens a woman's desire; some say, in fact, that it might have precisely the opposite effect.

A well-studied herb, agnus castus appears to work by evening out hormone imbalances that occur during the menstrual cycle. Specifically, it influences the pituitary gland to stem secretion of the hormone prolactin. When prolactin is reduced, an irregular menstrual cycle usually normalizes. This makes agnus castus useful for women who, month after month, experience premenstrual syndrome, menstrual cramps and menstrual irregularities.

During menopause, agnus castus is recommended for flooding, spotting, severe hot flushes and dizziness. Acne caused by menopausal changes might also be relieved with agnus castus.

Taken as a tea or tincture (sometimes called an extract), agnus castus is a slow-acting herb, so use it regularly for several months to reap its benefits. While it is generally regarded as safe, you should know that agnus castus may counteract the effectiveness of birth control pills.

Angelica sinensis

Botanical Name: *Angelica sinensis*

One of the first Chinese drugs mentioned in ancient medical books, Angelica sinensis (also known as Chinese angelica or dong quai) dates back to 400 BC and is the most popular of all Chinese herbs, especially for women.

In traditional Chinese medicine, doctors treat allergies, arthritis, nervousness and high blood pressure with Angelica sinensis, and they believe the herb has the power to prevent cancer. Because it's also believed that it helps a woman retain her youthful glow long past her youth, Angelica sinensis is an ingredient in Chinese beauty creams.

Angelica sinensis contains vitamins B_{12} and E and other active components, including ferulic acid, which eases menstrual cramps, muscle spasms and other types of pain. Its B_{12} content, along with folate and biotin, stimulates the formation and development of red blood cells in the bone marrow, effectively remedying a type of anaemia that commonly accompanies menstrual problems.

Herbalists report that Angelica sinensis regulates menstruation, eases cramps, relaxes the uterus, clears up psoriasis and eczema, reduces hot flushes and eases vaginal dryness. Angelica sinensis root can be taken in the form of tea or a tincture (sometimes called an extract) or in capsules. If you are still menstruating, herbalists recommend that you stop taking this herb one week before your period and resume at the end of your period.

Black Cohosh

Botanical Name: *Actea racemosa*

Also known as black snakeroot, bugbane and rattleroot, black cohosh was introduced to early settlers by Native Americans and comes from the Algonquin word *cohosh*, meaning 'knobby, rough roots'. Native American women traditionally relied on black cohosh for 'women's diseases'.

By the 1800s, herbal healers became convinced that black cohosh was a panacea and used it to treat everything from snakebite to smallpox to hypochondria. By 1912, black cohosh was one of the medicinal herbs most frequently prescribed by American doctors.

Black cohosh supplies oestrogenic sterols and glycosides (chemicals that help the body produce and use a variety of hormones) and a host of micronutrients. According to Commission E, the expert panel that judges the safety and effectiveness of herbal medicines for the German government, black cohosh is effective for treating PMS, painful menstruation and problems associated with menopause. In fact, studies indicate that it can be as effective as hormone replacement therapy for relieving hot flushes and other menopausal difficulties.

Black cohosh can be taken in the form of a decoction or a tincture (sometimes called an extract) or in capsules. Commission E recommends that black cohosh not be used for more than six months.

Cramp Bark

Botanical Name: *Viburnum opulus*

Although the bright red berries of the cramp bark bush are so bitter that birds won't touch them, humans have found a number of ingenious uses for them. Siberians distil cramp bark berries into a soul-warming brew, and Canadians substitute them for cranberries in jam or sauce.

For women, the bark of the cramp bark has another, far more useful purpose: for 700 years, this herb has been prescribed as a remedy for menstrual cramps, threatened miscarriage and pelvic pain, among other problems.

Also known as guelder rose, high cranberry and red, rose or water elder, cramp bark is closely related to black haw (*V. prunifolium*). Even under a microscope, the two plants appear identical. (For muscle spasm pain, however, cramp bark seems to be stronger than black haw.)

Cramp bark contains chemicals called hydroquinones, which have various medicinal actions, including one that combats heavy menstrual bleeding. It also contains scopoletin, which fights pain and muscle spasms and relaxes the uterus. Cramp bark is rich in valerianic acid, which has a relaxing effect on the reproductive organs.

Modern herbalists still consider cramp bark one of the best treatments for menstrual cramps. They also recommend it for heavy menstrual bleeding and menopausal flooding, as well as for tension headaches. The dried bark, which is generally regarded as safe, is usually decocted into a tea or made into a tincture (sometimes called an extract).

Ginseng

Botanical Names: *Panax ginseng* (Asian ginseng); *P. quinquefolium* (American ginseng)

Given that its common names also include 'root of life' and 'a dose of immortality', it's little surprise that ginseng has enjoyed a near-mythical reputation for thousands of years. This sweet and faintly aromatic root occupied a place of honour in China's 2,000-year-old medical manual *The Herbal Classic of the Divine Ploughman*. Today ginseng is still widely employed by Asians to rejuvenate themselves, increase sexual desire and ease difficult childbirth, among other uses. Native Americans relied on American ginseng for menstrual problems, headaches, exhaustion, fever, colic, vomiting and earaches.

Growing in popularity in the West is Siberian ginseng, which is not a true form of ginseng but the root of a plant called *Eleutherococcus senticosus*, which shares certain properties with true ginseng.

Ginseng root contains a banquet of active ingredients, including at least 18 different hormone-like saponins called ginsenosides, which botanists say fight stress and fatigue, protect the liver and guard against memory loss. Proponents say this herb can be of special help to women by relieving stress-related hot flushes at menopause and easing exhaustion during childbirth.

The age-old methods of using ginseng were to chew the root and to make it into a tea. Ginseng, however, is now also commonly taken in the form of capsules, tablets and liquid extracts. Experts recommend that to avoid irritability, you avoid consuming caffeine and other stimulants while using ginseng.

Lady's Mantle

Botanical Name: *Alchemilla vulgaris*

With its grey-green leaves and lacy blooms, lady's mantle has a long history of use as a 'women's herb'. The plant may have first been associated with women because the leaves resemble a woman's old-fashioned cloak. Other common names include ladies mantle, lion's foot and bear's foot.

In any case, as early as the 1600s, lady's mantle was used as an aid to conception, a miscarriage preventive and – of all things – a folk remedy for sagging breasts. The herb was also used to heal wounds and stop vomiting, diarrhoea and excess bleeding – uses that continue to this day.

Evidence suggests that plant compounds known as tannins, which are found in the leaves and flowers, make lady's mantle an effective, astringent remedy for closing and healing wounds and, when taken internally, for bleeding and diarrhoea.

In its review of scientific literature on lady's mantle, Commission E, the expert panel that judges the safety and effectiveness of herbal medicines for the German government, recommended it for mild diarrhoea that lasts only a few days.

Herbalists believe the astringent properties of lady's mantle work internally, making it an excellent choice for normalizing heavy periods and bleeding due to fibroid tumours. Herbalists say that lady's mantle also improves poor uterine tone, eases menopausal hot flushes and soothes mild menstrual aches and pains. It may also be used during pregnancy to allay morning sickness.

Generally regarded as safe to use, this herb is usually taken as a tea or tincture (sometimes called an extract). It's also sometimes applied externally as a herbal wash or poultice.

Liquorice

Botanical Name: *Glycyrrhiza glabra*

Liquorice is a grand old herb. Favoured in China for more than 5,000 years, its intensely sweet, fibrous root is still prescribed by herbalists for respiratory and digestive problems, and it is frequently used to heighten the effects of other herbs. In seventeenth-century England, liquorice was boiled with figs to quieten coughs and chest pains, and steeped in teas to relieve constipation and fevers. In fact, liquorice has been found in women's herbal formulas for hundreds of years, perhaps because it contains oestrogen-like compounds.

If you suck on a slice of dried liquorice root, your taste buds will quickly encounter this plant's most active compound: glycyrrhizin, a saponin that's 50 times sweeter than sugar. (Little wonder, then, that one of its other common names is sweet wood.) Structured like your body's hormones, glycyrrhizin may have a mild oestrogen-like effect, making it valuable for regulating hormones at menopause, according to herbalists and scientists.

Researchers have also found that compounds in liquorice have anti-inflammatory, anti-allergic and anti-arthritic actions. It is also used to ease coughs, clear respiratory congestion, soothe the digestive system and promote elimination.

While liquorice is usually taken medicinally as tea, experts advise against using it daily for more than four to six weeks. Overuse can lead to water retention, high blood pressure caused by potassium loss, or impaired heart and kidney function. You should also use this herb with caution if you are at risk of high blood pressure or water retention. If you have been diagnosed with diabetes, high blood pressure, liver or kidney disorders, or low potassium levels, avoid using liquorice altogether.

Motherwort

Botanical Name: *Leonurus cardiaca*

One old herbal text describes motherwort as powerful protection against wicked spirits – and indeed it has been used for thousands of years to dispel doldrums and anxiety.

With its dull green leaves and purplish blooms, this ancient herb 'makes mothers joyful and settles the womb, therefore it is called Motherwort', according to seventeenth-century English apothecary Nicholas Culpeper. Other common names include mother herb, heart heal, lion's tail and lion's ear.

A heart remedy throughout Europe and Asia, bitter-tasting motherwort was used in China to lengthen life. (Legend has it that a daily cup of motherwort tea helped one wise man live to see his 300th birthday.) The Greeks and Romans relied on it to cure all manner of physical and emotional problems.

Motherwort's leaves and flowers contain leonurine and stachydrine, alkaloids (or plant compounds) that herbalists say promote menstrual bleeding and the uterine contractions that lead to childbirth. The herb also contains bitter glycosides, mild sedatives and relaxants that may temporarily lower blood pressure.

Herbalists today use motherwort for a wide variety of 'women's conditions'. It soothes the stress of premenstrual syndrome and menopausal hot flushes. Evidence shows that it can also restore cardiac health and regulate a rapid heartbeat brought on by anxiety.

Motherwort is taken as a tea or tincture (sometimes called an extract). If you use it for tension relief, it may take about 15 minutes before you feel the effects.

Oat straw

Botanical Name: *Avena sativa*

A traditional staple of northern European diets, oats have been cultivated since at least 100 BC. While oats were prized as a stomach-satisfying grain, tea brewed from the herb's dried, pale green stems, leaves and grain husks (or straw) was and still is a common folk remedy for nervous exhaustion and sleeplessness. Historically, a good soak in an oat straw bath was said to relieve arthritis and rheumatism, among other problems.

In the nineteenth and early twentieth centuries, the plant ranked among the best restoratives for exhaustion brought on by a fever and for headaches associated with overwork or depression.

Herbalists report that tension headaches, insomnia, nervous exhaustion and that 'frazzled' feeling respond well to oat straw, which is regarded as a tonic that can relieve both physical and emotional fatigue as well as depression. Oat straw contains calcium and silicic acid (a component of silica), reportedly making this herb a good tonic for hair, nails and bones.

Herbalists say that drinking a few cups of oat straw tea every day can increase strength and energy and foster a feeling of calm. It's also believed that oat straw may encourage sweating and help remedy colds. In addition, it may sometimes be used to fight yeast infections.

This herb is taken as a tea or tincture (sometimes called an extract) or used as a healing wash for skin conditions. Because oat straw contains gluten, however, you shouldn't ingest it if you have gluten intolerance (coeliac disease).

Red Clover

Botanical Name: *Trifolium pratense*

Less than a century ago, red clover was the star ingredient in homemade spring tonics and commercial health tonics alike (including a concoction called Compound Number 7), thanks to its reputation as an all-around wellness herb and blood purifier.

The Chinese revered red clover sap as a remedy for colds and influenza. A popular healing plant in England and Germany, it travelled across the Atlantic with colonists and settlers in North and South America, where it grows wild today. At the turn of the last century, the herb was typically brewed into a strong tea to halt spasmodic coughing. Mennonite communities still rely on it to ease whooping cough and croup. This herb is also known as purple clover and meadow trefoil.

Herbalists report that red clover brings on a normal menstrual cycle, promotes fertility, balances hormones at menopause when menstrual periods are irregular, calms restlessness, soothes coughing and eases eczema and psoriasis. Apparently, the blossoms contain hormone-like substances called oestrogenic plant sterols. In addition, red clover has important vitamins and minerals, including calcium, magnesium, potassium and vitamins B and C. To make a red clover tea, soak the flowers in cool water overnight to extract the most minerals.

Vitamins and Other Supplements

Vitamins and supplements are not magic pills. But it can be really tempting to think of them that way. Anything that can help you ease menopausal symptoms *and* live longer, look younger, boost your energy levels and stave off cancer, depression and heart disease certainly sounds miraculous or magical.

Of course, they can't cure everything. But they can do a lot. And while the reasons for taking vitamins and other nutritional supplements are now based on solid science, shopping for them is still nothing less than overwhelming – letters and numbers, capsules and tablets, row upon row of bottles in different sizes and colours covered with enticing claims that compete for your attention and precious consumer spending power.

To sort through the confusion, we've put together this simple guide of seven nutritional supplements you should consider having on hand.

Calcium

By now, it's common knowledge that calcium plays an important role in the prevention of osteoporosis. What is less commonly known is that calcium plays an important role in treating high blood pressure, insomnia and menstrual and muscle cramps.

Yet calcium comes in so many forms, even as a supplement, that choosing among the varieties may be confusing. Here's a clue. When you're reading labels, look for the 'elemental calcium' listing to tell you how much you're really getting, says Dr Robert E. C. Wildman, a professor of nutrition. Most labels include this listing, he adds.

If the label does not indicate how much elemental calcium is in each tablet, you can use the table below. If you're taking a 500-milligram tablet of calcium carbonate, for example, you can see that it contains 40 per cent elemental calcium – which translates into 200 milligrams of calcium from each tablet. Here are the typical percentages of actual calcium in supplement products.

SUPPLEMENT	ELEMENTAL CALCIUM (%)
Calcium carbonate	40
Dicalcium phosphate	38
Bonemeal	31
Oyster shell	28
Dolomite	22
Calcium citrate	21
Calcium lactate	13
Calcium gluconate	9

You don't absorb all of the elemental calcium that's in a tablet, Dr Wildman points out – only 30 to 40 per cent (in fact, calcium citrate-malate, which is available mostly in fortified orange juice, is perhaps the best-absorbed form). If you take a supplement with food, a tablet of calcium carbonate is the most efficient way to get what you need. With supplements like calcium citrate, lactate or gluconate, you'll need to take more tablets to equal the amount of calcium in a single dose of calcium carbonate.

Aim for between 1,200 and 1,500 milligrams a day if you are over age 50 (1,000 milligrams if you're not quite there). And to get the most calcium from your supplements, divide your daily dose into two smaller doses, no more than 500 milligrams each. If you use calcium citrate, lactate or gluconate, you can take it between meals without absorption problems, and it also won't interfere with absorption of iron and other trace minerals. All other forms of supplemental calcium are best absorbed when taken with food. Avoid taking supplements at the same time as large amounts of wheat bran. Bran will move the supplements through your system before they can be absorbed.

To further aid absorption, get 400 IU of vitamin D daily from sunlight, fortified foods or supplements; it's not necessary to take the calcium and vitamin D together.

Good food sources of calcium include milk and other low-fat dairy products, sardines (with bones), kale and calcium-fortified juices.

Fibre

Worried about gaining weight as you go through menopause? Then pay attention to your fibre intake. Fibre is the indigestible part of all plant foods, including fruit, vegetables, grains and beans. It is not found in meat or any other animal foods.

Most fibre-rich foods contain both soluble and insoluble fibre. Soluble fibre dissolves in water in your intestinal tract, forming a glue-like gel. It softens stools and slows down stomach emptying, allowing for better digestion and helping you feel fuller longer, an effect that may aid weight loss.

But if you're like most Westerners, you're probably not getting enough. The typical diet includes only 10 to 15 grams of dietary fibre a day, but the recommended intake in the UK is 18 grams. However, cancer specialists believe that 35–40 grams is more like the quantity most of us should be eating. The current daily intake for most Australians is 20–25 grams, on average, well short of the 30–35 grams recommended by Nutrition Australia. More than half of the population of New Zealand consumes less than the recommended daily intake of 25–30 grams of fibre per day. For many of us, that means we need to double our current intake.

As far as the other health benefits that fibre provides, some studies have shown a link between high-fibre diets and a decreased risk of colon and breast cancers. Studies also have shown that people who get the most fibre in their diets are less likely to have heart disease.

To boost your fibre intake, health experts generally recommend that you get your fibre from food, not supplements. Switch from processed and fast foods to whole foods, including whole grains, fresh vegetables, fruit and beans, and you get not only a healthy dose of fibre but also a host of other nutrients that supplements don't provide.

Sometimes, though, we can't or won't get all the fibre we need. And that's when supplements can help. Whether you're adding more fibre-rich foods to your diet or taking fibre supplements, you need to increase your intake gradually. Since fibre isn't absorbed, it can ferment in the intestine, causing gas, bloating, cramps and diarrhoea.

And if you choose to use fibre supplements, always drink at least 240 ml (8 fl oz) of water with every dose. Fibre acts like a sponge, and if you don't drink plenty of fluids, it can swell and block part of the gastrointestinal tract.

Too much fibre can also block the absorption of vital minerals such as iron, calcium and zinc. And in some situations, it could also cause calcium losses.

If you supplement, try to get your fibre from a variety of sources in addition to a high-fibre diet. Look for products like psyllium, apple and grapefruit pectin, guar gum, methylcellulose and calcium polycarbophil. At your local healthfood shop, you may also find wheat and oat bran tablets and multifibre tablets with ingredients such as beet and carrot fibres.

Psyllium is a popular and inexpensive fibre supplement that can act as a laxative and lower cholesterol, says Dr William D. Nelson, a naturopathic doctor. This supplement is available in tablet, capsule and powder forms. All are equally effective, but fibre capsules and tablets are more expensive than powders.

Psyllium causes gas and bloating in some people. If that happens to you, try flaxseed, which is easiest to take in capsules or in powdered form. In addition to fibre, flaxseed contains lignans, compounds that may have anti-cancer, anti-bacterial, anti-fungal and anti-viral effects, says Dr Nelson.

Be wary, however, of marketing claims that fibre supplements containing chitosan (a form of chitin, which is a component of the shells of shellfish) promote weight loss, says naturopathic doctor Jennifer Brett. 'I've never seen any evidence that it works for weight loss,' she says. Even if chitosan did remove fat from the body as its proponents claim, it would also bind with and remove fat-soluble vitamins that your body needs, she says.

Animal studies have shown that chitosan can absorb LDL cholesterol (the bad type) and reduce lipid concentrations, but further studies are needed to confirm any cholesterol-lowering action. As for a weight-loss effect, some animals in the studies actually gained weight when they were fed chitosan, while others lost.

Flaxseed

If you're living with hot flushes, you may have been steadily filling your cupboard with linen clothes, that cool staple of summer wardrobes that are made from flax. According to researchers, you'd be wise, too, to add some flax to your plate. Recent studies have turned up some pretty convincing evidence that in addition to cooling hot flushes, flaxseed and flaxseed oil may improve heart health, fight breast and colon cancers, and boost the immune system.

Flaxseed is the richest source of alpha-linolenic acid (ALA), a plant source of omega-3 fatty acids, which are one of two families of essential fatty acids that the body needs but cannot make on its own. Omega-3s are the building blocks of eicosanoids, hormone-like compounds that regulate blood pressure, clotting and other body functions.

Plus, these small brown seeds hold some big promise for combating breast and colon cancers. In animal studies, flaxseed has significantly reduced existing breast and colon tumours while stopping new ones from getting started. In one study, researchers at the University of Toronto were able to reduce tumour size by more than half in animals that were fed flaxseed over a seven-week period. Flaxseed and flaxseed oil reduced the growth of existing tumours, but a component of flaxseed, called lignans, appeared to help prevent the development of new ones.

Lignans are plant-based compounds that can block oestrogen activity in cells, reducing the risk of certain cancers. Many plants have some lignans, but flaxseed has at least 75 times more than almost any other plant.

Lignans are phyto-oestrogens, meaning that they are similar to but weaker than the oestrogen that a woman's body produces naturally. Therefore, they may also help alleviate menopausal discomforts such as hot flushes and vaginal dryness. They are also anti-bacterial, anti-fungal and anti-viral.

Flaxseed also appears to reduce the risk of heart disease and stroke. One way that ALA helps the heart is by decreasing the ability of platelets to clump together, a reaction involved in the development of atherosclerosis (hardening of the arteries). ALA also lowers levels of dangerous LDL cholesterol and helps the body rid itself of blood fats called triglycerides, which at high levels can also be harmful to heart health.

Flaxseed oil comes in liquid and gelatine capsules, but you may want to skip the oil and just add flaxseed to your diet. The oil contains only trace amounts of the cancer-protective lignans because they are removed during processing.

Flaxseed is also an excellent source of fibre, whereas the oil has virtually none. As little as a handful of ground flaxseed contains six grams of fibre – as much as a large bowl of porridge. Grind whole seeds in your electric coffee grinder or food processor and sprinkle them on cereal, add them to smoothies or mix them with yoghurt or porridge oats. You can store whole seeds in a cool, dry cupboard for up to a year. Use any ground flaxseed immediately or keep it in the freezer, says Dr Diane Morris, a nutritionist. If you choose to use flaxseed oil, try substituting it for salad dressings instead of vegetable, olive or other oils. Never cook with flaxseed oil because it degrades quickly when exposed to heat and light. And remember to refrigerate it between uses.

To avoid weight gain, be sure to take the high calorie content of oil into account when figuring your daily calorie intake.

SAM-e

Because oestrogen levels seem to affect levels of serotonin, the feel-good hormone that helps make us feel mellow and more flexible in how we react to life's ups and downs, the sudden drop in oestrogen at menopause can have a profound effect on some women. So imagine a natural supplement that could relieve that depression faster than prescription drugs, as well as the pain of osteoarthritis.

Sound too good to be true? A nutritional supplement that has been used in Europe for years to treat depression has found its way to wider markets, and its benefits look promising. S-adenosylmethionine – or SAM-e (pronounced 'sammy') for short – promises to work faster than most prescription antidepressants, without the side-effects. SAM-e occurs naturally in your body and helps in the production of mood-lifting serotonin. Usually, your body can produce all the SAM-e it needs – but depressed women seem to make less SAM-e, so the theory goes that by taking supplements to raise levels to normal, your body follows suit by restoring its serotonin levels as well.

Experts say that you can use SAM-e with antidepressant drugs, or alone for mild to moderate depression, under your doctor's supervision. The usual dosage is 400 milligrams a day, but dosages up to 1,600 milligrams are safe. People who have bipolar disorder should be especially careful about using SAM-e because any kind of antidepressant can tip them over into a state of mania.

Look for enteric-coated capsules to protect your stomach from irritation; they keep the medicine from dissolving before it reaches your small intestine. Also, SAM-e has a better chance of working if you're getting adequate amounts of folate and vitamins B_{12} and B_6 to help the SAM-e along.

Vitamin C

In addition to abating menopausal discomforts such as heavy menstrual bleeding, vitamin C plays an important role in helping your body fight off a host of other conditions, including colds, angina, depression, heart disease and chronic inflammatory diseases such as lupus and rheumatoid arthritis.

While the RNI, the amount you need to take to stave off disease, is a modest 40 milligrams a day, some doctors recommend so-called megadoses of vitamin C, amounts far higher than the RNI, to flood the body with the vitamin during certain illnesses.

The thinking is that many illnesses, including heart disease, involve damage from free radicals, unstable molecules that affect healthy cells. Once it gets started, the damage can cause a chain reaction that quickly depletes inflamed tissue of vitamin C and allows the damage to spread even more.

While there is some research to indicate that taking additional vitamin C can help shorten the duration of a cold, there is little evidence to support the use of large amounts for illnesses such as glandular fever, hepatitis, cancer or AIDS, says Dr Balz Frei, professor of biochemistry and biophysics and director of the Linus Pauling Institute. 'I'm not saying that it doesn't work or that the theory behind this isn't sound. I'm saying that there is currently not enough scientific evidence to conclude that mega-doses of vitamin C provide health benefits beyond those of more moderate doses of the vitamin,' he says.

While vitamin C is considered generally safe at a wide range of dosages, getting more than 1,000 milligrams a day can cause diarrhoea; if this occurs, cut back until the diarrhoea stops. And if you're taking a high dosage, cut back to 100 milligrams at least three days before a physical examination or medical tests, as high amounts can interfere with some tests, including those for blood in the stool and for sugar in the urine. Large dosages may also affect anticoagulants (blood thinners).

If you'd rather stick to the vitamins you can get from food, good sources of vitamin C include broccoli, brussels sprouts, cabbage, chilli peppers, citrus fruit, guavas, mangoes, kale, parsley, red and green peppers and strawberries.

Vitamin D

Open just about any nutrition textbook to the pages on vitamin D, and you'll see haunting photographs of children with rickets, a deficiency condition. Their heads are large because their skull bones haven't fused properly, and their legs are bowed because their bones are too soft to support their weight.

Rickets is no longer common in the West, but vitamin D deficiency may play a contributing role in the development of osteoporosis, a condition of vital importance to women approaching menopause. The body needs a sufficient amount of vitamin D to make calcium and phosphorus available in the blood that bathes the bones. As these essential minerals are deposited, the bones mineralize, or harden. When blood levels of vitamin D are low, the rate of bone loss accelerates.

Bones aren't the only parts of our bodies that vitamin D befriends. Researchers are finding more and more places where it's active. Forms of vitamin D are being studied in the laboratory for the treatment of breast, prostate and colon cancers, plus a deadly skin cancer, melanoma. One form of vitamin D, as a topical cream named calcipotriol (Dovonex), showed marked improvement of psoriasis for up to 70 per cent of the people who used it.

The irony is that vitamin D is an essential nutrient that our bodies can make on any reasonably sunny day. In fact, it's called the sunshine vitamin because we can make all we need if we have enough sunlight hitting our skin. Nonetheless, vitamin D deficiency remains a real problem in the West, and it becomes increasingly likely in people aged 50 and older. As we age, our bodies don't manufacture the vitamin as easily. Plus, people just don't get enough of the few foods that contain vitamin D: milk and fatty fish such as mackerel and salmon.

'Most older people, especially those who use sunscreen, probably don't get enough sun to meet their vitamin D requirements,' says Dr Michael Holick, an endocrinologist. Nevertheless, it is possible to get an adequate amount of vitamin D from sunlight, he says. Dr Holick recommends that you expose your hands, face and arms to sunlight in the mid-morning or afternoon. If you live in northern Europe you'll have enough exposure if you get five to 15 minutes of sunlight three times a week in spring, summer and autumn. Winter sun isn't strong enough to meet your needs for vitamin D unless you live in sunny climes.

Fortunately, supplements are another reliable way to get what you need if you're not getting enough vitamin D from dairy sources or sunlight. You can take a multivitamin/mineral supplement that offers the RNI for women over 50 of 10 mcg of vitamin D.

The National Research Council, which sets standard, official guidelines for US health agencies, recommends a daily dosage of 600 IU for people over 70. Some studies show that people over 65 benefit from getting up to 800 IU a day, especially during the winter months.

Vitamin E

Vitamin E apparently has only one major role in the body, but that one is a whopper. 'It functions as our bodies' major fat-soluble antioxidant,' says Dr Maret Traber, an associate professor of nutrition. Vitamin E is found throughout our bodies in the tissues that contain fat, including in the protective membranes surrounding cells and in their nuclei, which contain the genetic material.

Vitamin E helps neutralize molecular particles called free radicals that are produced as a normal part of reactions that involve oxygen. 'A free radical is a molecule that has an unpaired electron, making it unstable,' Dr Traber says. Because the imbalance makes it 'hungry' for an electron, it steals one from some other molecule.

Unfortunately, that means that another molecule is short of an electron, so it becomes a free radical, which in turn strives to pluck an electron from some other unlucky molecule nearby. The effect is a chain reaction of free radical damage, kind of like a game of tag that's wildly out of control.

This game leads to trouble. When free radicals attack, cell membranes are damaged, sometimes beyond repair. If the cell contents leak out, the cell dies. Or, if the damage occurs in the membranes inside a cell, the cell's genetic material is harmed. If the membrane of the cell's power plant, the mitochondria, is damaged, trouble multiplies like a brawl at a football match. Free radicals normally generated inside the mitochondria leak out into the cell, and the resulting unrest spreads like wildfire.

Vitamin E can stop all this by donating one of its own electrons to a free radical. When that happens, there's no chain reaction. Vitamin E stops the outbreak of electron grabbing dead in its tracks. You could think of it as the referee at that rowdy game of football.

If you go by the research, even an exemplary diet can't give us the amounts of vitamin E that studies suggest provide protection from heart disease or enhance immunity. There is no RNI for vitamin E, but estimates of an optimal dosage really start at around 100 IU. You'd have to ingest 10.5 kg (23 lb) of boiled spinach, 900 g (2 lb) of peanuts, 360 ml (12 fl oz) of corn oil, or 3 tablespoons of wheatgerm oil to get close to that amount.

If you are watching your weight and reducing the amount of fat in your diet, you are even less likely to get close to the required amount of vitamin E. In one study of people who had cut their fat intake below 30 per cent of calories, daily vitamin E intake dropped from 14.5 to 9.5 IU.

While some researchers recommend getting 100 to 400 IU a day, a number of clinicians recommend even higher amounts for people aged 45 and older and for those with chronic diseases. One study, from researchers at the University of Texas, found that 400 IU a day was the minimum dosage of vitamin E required to significantly reduce LDL oxidation – a process that may contribute to heart disease by thickening and stiffening artery walls. Dosages up to 1,200 IU provided additional benefits. Taking 200 IU a day did not significantly reduce LDL oxidation, researchers found. Given this wide range of results, many experts are involved in ongoing discussions about new guidelines for recommending vitamin E.

THE ALTERNATIVE ROUTE: HEALING MODALITIES

The attraction of alternative practitioners is that they typically offer compassionate attention to your overall well-being. And because, according to its proponents, the focus of alternative medicine is preventive, it can help you avoid menopausal health problems altogether. But should the need arise, you can also expect an alternative practitioner to offer a unique array of gentle, drug-free methods to try to relieve your symptoms. Unlike the approach of conventional medicine, you can expect your remedies from an alternative health practitioner to be a highly personalized programme based on your individual symptoms, history and desires. Practitioners typically include their patients in decisions about what treatments fit since they traditionally value the roles that both mind and spirit play in the healing process.

Be alert when reading this section as to which particular methods appeal to you. Are you drawn to breath work to ease hot flushes? Are you interested in visiting a doctor of oriental medicine to ease heavy menstrual bleeding? Or are you intrigued by the idea of a yoga instructor teaching you ancient poses that lessen depression and anxiety? If you are still unsure of where to start, your best bet is to visit a naturopathic doctor (see 'Naturopathy' on page 284). These practitioners are skilled in the widest variety of natural therapy options. And for more information on these and other healing alternatives, visit:

• The Complementary Healthcare Information Service – UK, at *www.chisuk.org.uk*

CHINESE MEDICINE

What prompts women to give traditional Chinese medicine a try? Usually, some kind of chronic pain, says Barbara Bernie, president of the American Foundation of traditional Chinese medicine (TCM).

'Although we don't have statistics on how many people visit TCM practitioners, experience tells me that many people first try acupuncture, one of TCM's therapeutic treatments, for chronic pain that hasn't responded to traditional Western medicine.'

But traditional Chinese medicine is much more than the practice of acupuncture. It is a medical system that combines acupuncture with the use of medicinal herbs, massage and dietary therapy. Practitioners also often recommend exercise, breathing disciplines and meditation in the form of qi gong and t'ai chi as part of an ongoing, holistic wellness programme.

And when it comes to women's health concerns, practitioners say that TCM can't be beaten. Though some of the TCM concepts seem decidedly exotic to Westerners, the fact is that they have withstood the test of time.

If you choose to look further into what this ancient system can do for you,

---

- The Better Health Channel – Australia, at *www.betterhealthchannel.com.au*
- New Zealand Health Information, at *www.nzhealth.net.nz*
- The Confederation of Complementary Health Associations of South Africa, at *www.cochasa.org.sa*

Acupuncture and Acupressure: Find Pain Relief and Fight Hot Flushes

Acupuncture and acupressure are two facets of traditional Chinese medicine that, according to ancient Chinese precepts, can help maintain good health by restoring the body's harmonious balance of chi (pronounced 'chee'), or vital energy.

Normally, chi flows freely along invisible internal channels, or 'meridians', that traverse the body. Stress, poor nutrition, injuries or lack of

your first traditional Chinese medicine visit is likely to be quite different from the medical appointments that you're used to. First of all, TCM uses methods of diagnosis completely different from those of Western medicine. The practitioner will do nothing more invasive than examine your tongue and take your pulse. And before she does anything else, the TCM practitioner will interview you (unlike a Western doctor, who may question you while you're up on the examining table). But be prepared to answer a lot more questions than you're used to being asked – some more personal and graphic than those that your family doctor usually asks.

Overall, the advantages of traditional Chinese medicine fit well with the disadvantages of Western medicine. TCM excels when you have diverse symptoms that don't form a coherent picture. In Western medicine you go to see specialists who treat your symptoms independently. For example, you might see an ear, nose and throat specialist for your sinus problems and a gastroenterologist for your stomach problems. A TCM practitioner would see all those symptoms as part of an overall pattern and would treat you accordingly. In fact, stomach disorders are especially well-suited to TCM.

exercise, however, can create obstructions in the meridians that keep chi from flowing freely. Like a stream that's been dammed, chi overflows in certain parts of the body but barely trickles into others. Such imbalance leads to weakness, and weakness can lead to disorder and render the body more susceptible to disease.

Acupuncture needles, inserted at certain 'acupoints' along the meridians, trigger healing because they break up obstructions, stimulate energy, or drain energy in a meridian, bringing the body back into balance and allowing chi to flow freely again. Of course, the needles need to be in the right spots in the correct meridians to do the trick. The right acupoint can be a distance from the ailing area.

The needles are so small that there usually isn't any bleeding, except in some areas with a lot of blood vessels, like the hands. (If you see an acupuncturist, make sure disposable needles are used to prevent transmission of blood-borne illnesses. Most acupuncturists use them.)

Acupressure is an offshoot of acupuncture. According to legend, acupuncture originated with China's Yellow Emperor and his ministers in 2500 BC. Historians, however, suspect that it evolved gradually. When the Chinese healers realized that they could achieve similar results simply by pressing on – rather than inserting needles into – specific points on the body, acupressure emerged as another way to stimulate healing.

Like acupuncture, acupressure is virtually free of side-effects. And though it isn't generally regarded as being as potent as acupuncture, it's something that patients can learn to use on their own.

What Acupuncture and Acupressure Can Do for You

While researchers have yet to explain in Western terms why acupuncture and acupressure work, the most widely accepted benefit of these treatments is pain relief. Controlled clinical studies have found acupuncture considerably more effective than placebo, or dummy, treatment in relieving pain. Many studies have divided patients into two groups: those who have had actual treatment (needles inserted at appropriate acupoints) and those who have had 'sham' acupuncture (needles inserted at the wrong places).

According to Dr Bruce Pomeranz, a neurophysiologist, professor at the University of Toronto School of Medicine, and one of the world's foremost acupuncture researchers, who has reviewed more than a dozen such studies, 55 to 85 per cent of patients who got the real thing reported relief from chronic pain, compared with just 35 per cent of those who received the placebo treatment.

Studies show that acupuncture can also help relieve nausea, whether it's the result of a turbulent car journey, chemotherapy or pregnancy. And other research suggests that acupuncture may help treat arthritis, asthma, bronchitis, cold symptoms, migraines, premenstrual syndrome and tennis elbow. It may also speed recovery from stroke, partially reverse nerve damage caused by diabetes, ease bladder problems, lessen depression, lower blood pressure, speed up labour, and relieve hot flushes during menopause.

Acupressure's tension-relieving potential may also explain its effect on pain and other symptoms. Numerous studies find that the body's own physiological response to stress – increased blood pressure and an out-pouring of adrenaline – can contribute to heart disease, depression, irritability, insomnia, headaches, difficulty concentrating, dampened immunity and other problems that often coincide with menopause.

Getting Started:
Self-acupressure for Good Health

You can learn simple self-acupressure techniques from a trained acu-pressurist or an acupuncturist, or from tapes or books.

Before you give it a try, here are a few pointers on proper technique and some caveats to keep in mind.

Get trim. Trim your nails before you start so that you don't dig into your skin.

Stick to the middle. Your middle finger is the longest and strongest and the best suited for self-acupressure. If it's not strong enough, try using your knuckles, your fist or the rubber on the end of a pencil, suggests Dr Michael Reed Gach, founder and director of the Acupressure Institute.

Tread carefully. Avoid applying acupressure to areas with scars, infections, ulcers or recent burns. Don't apply pressure directly over an artery or over the genitals. And go easy on the abdominal area. Touch, don't press, sensitive areas on the throat, below the ear, or on the outer breast near the armpit, according to Dr Gach. Also, if you have a serious or chronic illness, such as heart disease, cancer or high blood pressure, talk to your doctor and a professional acupressurist before using self-acupressure.

Don't eat and press. If you've just eaten a heavy meal, wait an hour before beginning an all-body regime, says Dr Gach. 'Many of the meridians cross the stomach, and if there's a lot of food in the stomach, the energy can get blocked, causing nausea.'

Zero in. Search for acupoints by carefully probing with your thumb. Acupoints are usually much more sensitive than the surrounding area, so be on the alert for sensitivity.

Make it hurt a little. One of the most common mistakes that novices make is to press too lightly. 'You have to press hard enough,' says Dr Pomeranz. 'Press until you get an aching sensation. A lot of people don't do that. They're too timid.'

AYURVEDA

Ayurveda is an approach to physical health, mental clarity and spiritual ful-filment that traces its roots to the essential religious texts of Hinduism. Imagine that one of the books of the Old Testament were a treatise on every practical detail of achieving physical, mental and emotional balance in order to perfect the individual's relationship with the Divine Power, and you'll have a sense of the breadth and depth of Ayurveda.

'The most important thing to know about Ayurveda is that it treats the whole person, not just the person's health problems,' says Robert E. Svoboda, an American who graduated from the Tilak Ayurveda Mahavidyalaya, an Ayurvedic school in Pune, India, and who now works with the Ayurvedic Institute. 'It isn't just about clearing up symptoms or even curing disease. It's also about restruc-turing the content of a person's consciousness so that he can be aware of the essential nature and meaning of life.'

One of the core ideas of Ayurveda is that the fundamental energy of life expresses itself through the three doshas – vata, pitta and kapha – which are basically three different types of constitutions. According to Ayurveda, your doshas are determined at the moment of conception, so every person has a dif-ferent mixture of doshas; usually, one dosha is predominant, and another is sec-ondary. Of course, the constitution you were born with is affected by day-to-day

---

Press your fingertips in firmly – at a 90-degree angle to the skin – exploring until you find the sensitive spot. Push hard but not to the point that you puncture the skin. Often you'll feel the same sensation that you get when you hit your funny bone – part pain, part numbness, part tingle. If you have well-developed muscles, you'll need to use deeper pressure. Women often need less pressure than men. Don't press any point that's excruciatingly painful. Acupressure should hurt a little, according to Dr Gach.

Make it last. Maintain pressure for 15 to 30 seconds per spot. Use a stopwatch or count 'one thousand and one, one thousand and two' to pace yourself. If you're working on a spot that has been injured or is painful or tense, hold it until the hurt lessens, but no more than five minutes, Dr Gach says. If you're just starting to use self-acupressure, don't work on the same spot more than two or three times a day. 'If you do more than that,

factors such as your work, the people you spend time with, and the foods you eat. Ultimately, the way to a healthy constitution is to keep your doshas balanced so that no single one becomes too active or too inactive.

In the West, there are few properly trained Ayurvedic practitioners as there are neither licencing procedures nor an accrediting board (although this is in the process of being rectified in the UK). If you're interested in exploring Ayurvedic therapies, your best bet is to choose a practitioner who combines Western medical training with Ayurvedic training or to coordinate Ayurvedic consultations with your regular doctor.

If you're not in the care of an Ayurvedic practitioner but would like to try out Ayurveda's healthcare philosophy, you can start your path towards mind–body healing with these simple lifestyle changes, which are part of the optimal Ayurvedic routine.

- Rise early – by 6 am, if possible.
- Meditate for at least 20 minutes once or twice each day.
- Keep your diet simple. A vegetarian or modified vegetarian diet is best. Make lunch the major meal of the day, and eat a light dinner early in the evening, preferably between 5 and 6 pm.
- Take short walks after meals to aid digestion.
- Get to bed early – ideally, by 10 pm.

you could release too much energy in that area, and this could create blockages in other places,' he says.

Do it daily. Make sure that you apply acupressure often enough to get results. Dr Pomeranz recommends doing your regime every day.

Alexander Technique: Improve Your Posture and Become More Aware of Yourself

Long before menopause, most of us start out with picture-perfect posture; as toddlers, we arrive with our heads up and our limbs loose. But as our bodies develop, we may slouch if we feel 'too tall' or hunch our shoulders to hide our chests. Later, we may succumb to fashion and wear high heels and carry heavy handbags that further distort our posture and movement. And it's precisely these types of poor posture habits that *can* affect your life – and your health, according to teachers of the Alexander Technique, a movement-training programme in which an instructor studies how you sit, stand, walk and bend in order to correct postural and tension-related mistakes and help you increase your awareness of how you might move more naturally.

Developed in the late 1800s by F. M. Alexander, a Shakespearean actor, the Alexander Technique helps you restore the effortless way of carrying yourself without compressing your spine, says Vivien Schapera, a teacher of the technique.

'The hallmark of the Alexander Technique is if a movement takes effort, it's wrong. What's causing you to slouch is the excessive unconscious contraction of muscles – in the stomach, the back, the shoulders – throughout your body,' she says. 'The Alexander Technique shows you how to free up your body so that you stop pulling on your skeleton with your habitually tense muscles.'

By taking stress off the body, the technique can help ease backaches, neck pains, joint problems, headaches, temporo-mandibular disorder, repetitive strain injuries and voice strain.

People commonly walk with the head pulled back and down on the neck. This compresses the joints and discs of the neck and back, and can lead to physical woes such as headaches, says Deborah Caplan, a physiotherapist and teacher of the Alexander Technique. 'The head weighs about 5.5 kg (12 lb), and the vertebrae at the top of the spine are very delicate,' she says. 'People should ask themselves, "Could I have less tension in my neck and shoulders?"'

What the Alexander Technique Can Do for You

An Alexander Technique instructor can teach you to be more fully aware of yourself when you're walking, standing, sitting and working. Your teacher will combine manual guidance and verbal instruction, and you will be able to apply what you learn in your lesson to your daily life. 'The technique is virtually impossible to learn to do on your own,' says Vivien Schapera.

The learning takes place in two ways, says Deborah Caplan. 'You learn as the principles are taught to you verbally by a teacher, and you learn on a kinesthetic level by the teacher gently guiding you with her hands into applying the correct use.'

Usually, the teacher puts her hand near your head and spine while you sit, stand or move. This helps remind you to keep your head easefully balanced on your spine and helps you maintain a non-compressing posture, says Judith Stern, a physiotherapist and expert in Alexander Technique.

Practitioners use mirrors to show you the difference between what you feel you're doing with your body and what you're really doing. It can be an eye-opening experience. For example, when your shoulder muscles relax, you might feel like you're slouching, but the mirror shows you standing effortlessly upright, says Vivien.

'The teacher guides you through everyday activities, such as sitting, bending, breathing and talking,' she says. 'If you were a musician, for example, I would ask you to bring in your instrument so that I could see what you do while you play.'

You'll also learn what Alexander Technique teachers call constructive rest, says Judith. You lie down on your back on the floor or a table, knees bent and feet flat on the surface, and learn to release excess muscle tension in your body.

'Allow your neck to release so that your head balances delicately on top of your spine, then allow your torso to release in length and width,' she says. 'Then you allow your legs to release from your torso and allow your arms to release from your torso.'

How many lessons will you need? While this varies from person to person, it usually takes at least 30 visits to make a lasting difference on your postural habits, and most experts recommend scheduling at least one lesson a week.

Getting Started: Balance Your Body

Here are a few hints from top Alexander Technique instructors about how to put your posture into tip-top form.

Kick off your heels. High-heeled shoes are an enemy to good posture because of the way they slant the foot and throw the body out of alignment, notes Deborah Caplan. Flats with cushioned soles give the best support.

'Walking in high heels jars the whole body,' she says. 'The foot is designed to absorb the shock of walking, but with heels the result is a tremendous amount of stress on the back.'

HOMOEOPATHY

Developed during the late eighteenth century by the German physician Samuel Hahnemann, homoeopathy (from the Greek words *homoeo*, meaning 'like', and *pathos*, meaning 'suffering') is based on the principle of similars. A substance that causes certain symptoms in a healthy person will *cure* those symptoms in a sick person.

Dr Hahnemann found that administering medicines that produced symptoms similar to those his sick patients were experiencing relieved his patients' suffering. However, the patients sometimes suffered ill-effects from the full-strength medicines. He therefore set about developing a method of making the medicines safer. After much experimenting, he found that diluting and shaking the medicines could enhance their healing effects while reducing their harmful effects. In fact, the more he diluted and shook, or succussed, the medicines, the more potent they became.

Modern homoeopathic remedies are *potentized*, meaning that a substance will be added to water, and then succussed 60 or more times. The mixture is then diluted again with water. The process can be repeated up to hundreds of times, until not a molecule of the original substance remains in the remedy.

The principle of potentized remedies gives even experienced homoeopaths pause when it comes to explaining how their healing art works. But on one thing they all agree – it does.

'The bottom line is that no one really knows how homoeopathic remedies work,' says Dr Linda Johnston, a homoeopath and founder of the Academy for Classical Homoeopathy. 'What I do know is that my patients get better. Unlike conventional medicine, homoeopathy doesn't treat symptoms – it corrects whatever is disturbing your system and producing those symptoms.'

For her female patients, some of homoeopathy's benefits include relief from menstrual and menopause difficulties. 'I think the fact that homoeopathy is

Unlock those legs. Perhaps more than men, women commonly cross their legs and hold the inner thighs together, which can lead to back problems because of a twist it creates in the lower spine and pelvis, notes Don Krim, chairman of the North American Society of Teachers of the Alexander Technique. 'They're often told to keep their legs together. But

---

non-toxic and has no side-effects makes it very helpful for women's health problems,' says Dr Johnston.

According to other experts, the real benefit of applying homoeopathy to the problems of menopause or PMS is that instead of taking a powerful drug on a regular basis, you can be given a remedy that you might take only a few times to regulate your system. The right remedy can end PMS symptoms entirely.

'Another plus is that unlike other approaches that have you stick to special routines or keep journals of your symptoms, homoeopathy doesn't require that women change their lifestyles to eliminate PMS,' says Dr Johnston. 'Instead, homoeopathy will correct the physiological problem that causes PMS in the first place.'

That doesn't necessarily mean that homoeopathy is the answer to everything. Homoeopathy might not be the appropriate solution for all the problems many women face around the time of menopause. Vaginal dryness, for example, doesn't usually respond well to homoeopathy. Plus, because each woman's menopausal problems present themselves differently, each woman needs a homoeopathic remedy individualized just for her.

Homoeopathic remedies may not look like any medicine that you've ever taken before. Don't be surprised, for example, if yours is a couple of dozen of pinhead-size sugar drops, to be downed all at once and just once. Remedies come in various concentrations, marked with a number and either a 'C', for the centesimal scale, which means potencies are diluted 100 times each time that they are shaken, or an 'X', for the decimal scale, which means that potencies are diluted 10 times each time that they are shaken. The higher the number, the more dilute the substance, yet the more powerful it is. Of the two units, C is more common. And with your medicine might come instructions to avoid coffee, mint toothpastes and strong-smelling substances such as camphor, eucalyptus and peppermint.

keeping your legs together as you move can distort the balance between the hip, knee and ankle joints, causing strain.'

Rather than pulling your knees together after you sit down, keep each knee lined up with your feet.

Sit up tall. Many working women spend their days slouched behind a computer, says Deborah. For good sitting posture, it's most important to have a chair that supports the lower back – one that's not so deep or high that your feet can't rest comfortably on the floor. 'Slouching undermines support of the spine and weakens the muscles, stretches the ligaments, and strains the facet joints in the back of the spine and the discs,' she says. 'Plus, the shoulders slip forward and put strain on the neck.' Try to avoid sitting in peculiar positions. Tucking one leg under the other might give you a sense of support, for example, but it actually causes the body to twist and contort, notes Vivien Schapera. It is ideal to sit with your feet apart and have them resting on an adjustable footrest or flat on the floor, which gives more support to the back.

Bend with care. When you reach down to pick something up, make sure that you're not just bending at the waist, says Judith. 'You should be bending over so that the hips, knees and ankles are doing the work,' she says. 'When you bend at your waist, the spine has no hinge joints at that point. It's a real strain because the back muscles aren't designed for that kind of work.'

Stand up for yourself. Long hours of sitting without a break are sure to aggravate posture problems, notes Vivien. 'All you need to do is stand up every 20 minutes or so and then sit back down again. Otherwise, your muscles get fatigued and have no choice but to tighten and collapse into themselves.'

Do some heady running. Most people jog with their heads back and down, says Judith. The result is that you end up pulling your head back rather than keeping it aligned with your torso and legs. 'Don't move your head in the opposite direction of your legs,' she says. 'Keep your head balanced and your spine lengthened.'

Don't hold the phone. If you're on the phone all day – especially if you're typing while talking – you harm your body by pressing the receiver to your shoulder, says Judith. Use a headset, to avoid spine compression and body contortion, she says.

Cue yourself to remember. Post notes reminding yourself to be aware of your posture, Judith suggests. 'You could stick a note on your computer that says, "Think". You'll start paying attention to how you're holding yourself: Are your legs relaxed? How are you breathing? Things like that,' she says.

Breath Work: Ease Hot Flushes and Restore Your Natural Calm

Most of us have forgotten how to breathe correctly. Proper breathing not only helps alleviate emotional problems but also helps soothe physical ones, like hot flushes, PMS, asthma and insomnia, according to advocates of the therapy known as breath work.

We're born breathing the right way, says Dr C. Shaffia Laue, a holistic psychiatrist. The right way to breathe is deep down in the abdomen. Watch a newborn's tummy slowly rise and fall with each inhalation and exhalation, and you'll see how it's done. Unfortunately, over time most of us unwittingly change from deep abdominal breathing to 'chest breathing', in which we hold our stomachs tight and breathe shallowly.

Shallow breathing spells trouble because it delivers less air per breath to our lungs. Less air per breath means that we take more frequent breaths, but this only makes matters worse, triggering a series of physiological changes that constrict our blood vessels.

'The end result of the whole process is that less oxygen reaches the brain, the heart and the rest of the body,' says Dr Robert Fried, a professor of psychology and author of *The Breath Connection*.

This undersupply of oxygen can leave us feeling dizzy, shaky, groggy and ill-equipped to make decisions. A chronic undersupply of oxygen can contribute to fatigue, depression, stress, anxiety and even panic attacks and phobias, explains Dr Laue.

Shallow chest breathing can also contribute to stress-related disorders such as PMS, menstrual cramps, headaches, migraines, insomnia, high blood pressure, asthma, back pain and allergies. And since rapid shallow breathing leads to the constriction of blood vessels, it can boost blood pressure and even trigger arterial spasms, says Dr Fried.

What Breath Work Can Do for You

What makes us switch from deep, satisfying abdominal breathing to shallow chest breathing in the first place? Stress, among other things, Dr Laue says.

When you're under stress, your diaphragm – the internal muscle between your chest and abdomen – contracts partway. This shrinks the space in your chest into which your lungs can expand, Dr Fried explains. Your breathing becomes shallow and rapid, your blood vessels contract, and you start selling yourself short on oxygen. Since rapid shallow breathing also contributes to stress, it creates a vicious circle. Stress leads to shallow breathing, which leads to stress, and so on.

Respiratory problems such as asthma can also trigger rapid shallow breathing, says Dr Fried. Since shallow breathing also exacerbates asthma, this, too, can start a cycle of asthma attacks, shallow breathing and more asthma attacks.

Getting Started: Breathing Lessons

Fortunately, most of us can relearn deep abdominal breathing by practising simple relaxation and breathing techniques.

'After people start abdominal breathing, they're less anxious, less depressed and less stressed, and they sleep better and have more energy,' says Dr Laue. Women approaching menopause may suffer less severe symptoms, too, once they start breathing abdominally.

The best way to learn how to breathe properly is to find a physiotherapist or psychotherapist who does breath work or a doctor who can teach you breathing exercises, watch you do them and correct any mistakes, says Dr Laue. Unfortunately, doctors and psychotherapists who use therapeutic breath work are few and far between. If you can't find one, a yoga, qi gong or martial arts teacher may be able to help you since abdominal breathing is an important part of those disciplines. Failing that, look for a good video, Dr Laue suggests.

If you have diabetes, low blood sugar or kidney disease, says Dr Fried, you should not practise breath work without your doctor's approval.

First, relax. Relax before practising abdominal breathing, and you'll find the job easier, Dr Laue says. She suggests the following progressive relaxation exercise. Though some therapists teach a progressive relaxation exercise that actually has you tense your muscles first, Dr Laue says that some people have a hard time relaxing their muscles after doing that. She prefers this version, in which you *imagine* tensing your muscles. Wear comfortable clothes for this exercise.

- Lie down.

- Starting at your feet and working up to your head, imagine tensing and then relaxing each part of your body.

- Imagine tensing your feet for four or five seconds; then imagine releasing the tension for four or five seconds.

- Moving up to your calf muscles, imagine tensing and relaxing those muscles. Imagine the wind blowing leaves along the gutter on a windy day. In your mind's eye, feel your breath moving the tension down your body and out the soles of your feet.

- Continue moving upward through your hips, abdomen, arms and chest. While you are focusing on your heart, imagine the sun melting the snow on an early-spring day. Feel the energy of the sun melting the tension in your body and then the tension running off your body like snow melting in spring sunshine.

- Continue with your shoulder, neck and head muscles, and end with your forehead. Finish by imagining yourself tensing and relaxing in a quiet place in nature where you feel very safe and peaceful.

Breathe by the book. Once you're relaxed, remain lying down and place a book on your abdomen. When you inhale, push the book upward, using your stomach muscles. When you exhale, pull the book downward with your stomach muscles. Make sure that your inhalations and exhalations are of equal duration, Dr Laue says. 'If you breathe out to a slow count of three, breathe in to a slow count of three.' Practise for 10 to 20 minutes twice a day, and eventually you'll be breathing from your abdomen automatically – even when you sleep, Dr Laue says.

NATUROPATHY

Naturopathy, also called naturopathic medicine, incorporates a wide range of alternative treatments – Ayurvedic medicine, botanical medicine, exercise therapy, homoeopathy, hydrotherapy, massage, meditation, nutritional therapy, osteopathy and traditional Chinese medicine. Doctors of naturopathy mix and match different treatments, customizing therapy for each individual woman and her particular health condition.

The way naturopaths see it, their job is to teach you how to *stay* healthy. Should you become ill, they're there to bolster your body's defences with the best that natural medicine has to offer.

'The conventional medical approach is basically: kill disease, kill disease, kill disease,' explains Dr Joseph Pizzorno Jr, founding president of Bastyr University of Naturopathic Medicine.

'The natural medicine approach is to help the person live healthier,' he says. 'While we may use therapies that have a direct impact on disease, we're much more interested in utilizing therapies that help support the body's natural healing processes, rather than those that take over the healing process of the body.'

Naturopaths don't reject conventional medicine out of hand, however. For acute health problems such as pneumonia and for life-threatening illnesses such as cancer, conventional medicine is still your best bet, says Dr Pizzorno. Naturopathic doctors, who use blood, urine and other standard medical tests in

Imagine. Imagery can also help you breathe correctly, says Nancy Zi, a classical opera singer, voice teacher, practitioner of qi gong and innovator of chi yi, a system of breathing exercises. Chi yi, she explains, is a cross between traditional Chinese qi gong breathing exercises and the breath training that professional singers get. Nancy suggests this simple exercise as a starter.

Imagine that your body is a giant upside-down eye dropper. Your mouth and nose are the dropper's opening, and your stomach is its bulb. With your hands on your stomach, breathe in deeply, imagining the air filling the bulb. Your stomach should expand when you do this. Then exhale, tightening your abdominal muscles as if squeezing the eye dropper bulb.

diagnosis, may refer patients with such problems to doctors or osteopaths. But naturopathic medicine is the ticket for chronic or less severe conditions that aren't life-threatening, he says.

Unfortunately, there aren't any scientific studies comparing naturopathy with conventional care. Even the best researchers would be hard-pressed to design such a study. Naturopathy includes so many therapies that controlling for all the variables would be virtually impossible.

The diversity in training results in a greater number of options, which is one of the big advantages of the naturopathic approach, naturopathic doctors say. In naturopathic medical school, students study anatomy, physiology, biochemistry, neurology, pathology and diagnostic techniques. In addition, they take courses in homoeopathy, therapeutic nutrition, hydrotherapy, botanical medicine, spinal manipulation and other therapeutic modalities rarely taught in conventional medical schools.

Disparate as they are, all naturopathic treatments share the same philosophy: help the body heal itself. And from the naturopathic perspective, symptoms of illness are also signs that the body is trying to heal itself. A rash, for example, is a sign that the body is trying to protect itself from an irritant. So according to the naturopathic approach, rather than override the body's attempts at healing – as when a person treats the rash by applying an anti-inflammatory cream – your best efforts should aim to gently enhance the body's own, natural healing efforts.

Yoga: Stretch Your Body and Ease Your Spirit

Started as a spiritual discipline 6,000 years ago in India, the practice of yoga has newly emerged as a powerful remedy for ailments such as menstrual cramps, rashes, mood swings and varicose veins, making it a valuable healing tool for women.

The term *yoga* comes from the Sanskrit word meaning 'to yoke' – that is, to join the mind and body together, says Dr Richard C. Miller, a yoga instructor and psychologist and co-founder of the International Association of Yoga Therapists. 'Some people interpret yoga as the union of different forces or energies,' he says.

The physical, spiritual and psychological aspects of yoga make it a useful therapy for health ailments, says Dr Carrie Angus, medical director for the Center for Health and Healing at the Himalayan International Institute of Yoga Science and Philosophy. Physically, yoga can build strength and improve flexibility because it stretches and strengthens the muscles, she says. It's good for the spine because it loosens the back and aids good posture, such as correcting slumped, rounded shoulders. Correcting posture mis-alignment helps free the rib cage, allowing you to breathe more deeply. And in addition to strengthening the body's ability to heal itself, yoga can coun-teract negative emotions such as anger, anxiety and depression, she adds.

'Doing yoga postures and concentrating on breathing is soothing and relaxing. And it gives you something else to focus on,' says John Orr, an instructor of physical education at Duke University, and formerly an ordained Theravadin Buddhist monk who practised in Thailand and India.

After people start doing yoga to relieve stress or physical problems, they gradually discover the deeper psychological benefits, says John. 'In spend-ing quiet time alone, you get to know yourself better. So yoga keeps you in touch with your physical, mental and spiritual self.'

The calm and well-being that yoga creates has been shown to counter that stress reaction, says Dr Lee Lipsenthal, medical director at the Pre-ventive Medicine Research Institute. 'What we find is that with yoga, heart disease begins to regress and blockages in the arteries shrink,' he notes. 'The goal is to get people to slow down, which in turn lowers their blood pressure and their heart rate.'

What Yoga Can Do for You

Women especially can benefit from yoga. It's claimed to ease the pain of PMS as well as help ease the discomforts of pregnancy, childbirth and certain changes associated with menopause, such as hot flushes. 'It is believed that breathing through your left nostril, for example, creates a cooling breath. This can be used to cool the system down and ease hot flushes,' says Dr Lipsenthal.

Also, evidence suggests that women who practise yoga are better off emotionally – less irritable and more congenial – than others. One study compared two groups: 12 women between the ages of 27 and 55 who did yoga postures, meditation and breathing exercises, and 13 women who had no experience with relaxation exercises and who didn't do yoga exercises. The women who practised yoga scored much better on self-tests designed to measure both positive emotions (such as euphoria) and negative emotions (such as excitability).

Although yoga has hundreds of poses, most routines contain about 20 different ones, with specific poses used to help specific ailments. Poses that emphasize sitting on the floor with your legs spread or lying on your back with your open legs up against a wall can ease cramps and PMS, for example, says Dr Angus. Poses that focus on your pelvis help direct energy to the area and ease menstrual problems, she adds. Bloating, for example, is said to be caused by stagnation of bodily fluids in the pelvic cavity. When you stretch that area, you get fresh blood pumping to the underlying muscles and tissues.

Getting Started: a Home Yoga Routine

Which routine of poses should you choose? It all depends on your physical problems, says Dr Miller. 'There would be a different one for women with back pain than for women with bladder problems,' he says. 'When teaching yoga, I always individualize the postures to each person in the class.' So the best strategy is to sign up for a class with an instructor you feel comfortable with.

Once you start practising yoga at home, follow these directives from expert instructors.

Get an early start. You can do yoga at any time of the day, but Dr Miller recommends doing it in the morning. 'The effect lasts eight to ten hours, so you can enjoy it for the rest of the day.'

Get comfortable. Using a mat, blanket, rug, cushion or chair, sit with your upper body erect but relaxed. Take a minute to check in mentally and put aside all the things that you've been thinking about.

Quiet your mind. Each yoga class begins and ends with a few minutes of meditation to quiet your mind, Dr Angus says. 'It's about focusing the mind on one thing, like your breath or a word such as *peace* or *love*. In that stillness, you can have all kinds of revelations about what you need in life and what's true for you.'

A quiet mind can help ease anxiety and depression. You come to realize that lots of things are uncontrollable and that you have to let go of what you can't control.

When clearing your mind for yoga, you should sit up either on the floor or in a chair, with your head, neck and trunk in a straight line, and take ten to 15 deep breaths, says Dr Angus.

Focus. Once your body starts to relax, focus on one sound or one object. 'For example, think "so" while you're breathing in and "hum" as you breathe out. It takes patience, so if you can do it for one minute, you're doing great,' says Dr Angus. With practice, you will be able to focus your mind for longer and longer periods.

Don't make it difficult. Although classes usually run for 60 to 90 minutes, a home yoga routine could be effective at 20 to 30 minutes, notes Dr Miller.

After doing deep breathing for two to three minutes, do varying yoga poses, synchronized with deep breathing, for about 15 minutes. Repeat this three days a week.

Don't push yourself. In yoga, the philosophy of 'no pain, no gain' just doesn't apply, says Dr Miller. 'Trying to do more than your body can handle is the way that people injure themselves,' he says. 'You should be listening to your body all the time.'

Chapter

10

STRAIGHT TALK ABOUT THE MENOPAUSE

T HE MENOPAUSE – AND THE YEARS BEFORE AND AFTER – CAN BE a confusing time, between the seemingly endless changes and the health worries that surround it. So here are the most commonly asked questions, with complete, detailed, up-to-the-minute answers from specialists such as Dr Mary Jane Minkin, an obstetrician-gynaecologist, clinical professor at Yale University School of Medicine, Dr Pamela M. Peeke, author of *Fight Fat after Forty*; and Toby Hanlon, a women's health expert.

Predicting the Menopause

Q: 'Is there a test that tells me if I'm menopausal and should be taking oestrogen replacement therapy?'

A: *Dr Minkin replies:* Tests measuring blood levels of oestradiol and follicle-stimulating hormone (FSH) are often used to gauge a woman's menopausal status. But neither test tells you absolutely whether you are menopausal or how far along in the process you are.

Why Tests Fall Short

The only sure way to confirm the menopause is by determining when you've gone 12 consecutive months without a menstrual period. If you've reached that point and are also having hot flushes, night sweats and sleep disturbances, you've probably reached menopause. I don't need a test to confirm that.

But what about a woman in her forties who is having irregular periods and hot flushes and suspects she's headed in the direction of menopause? I don't recommend testing oestradiol and FSH levels in this case. They are so variable from day to day and week to week in women approaching menopause that whatever levels you get on a particular day aren't necessarily conclusive. You'd have to repeat the test over time to get any valid results. And neither of these tests can tell you whether you're finished forever with your periods. (*A word of caution*: an elevated FSH and missed periods for three or four months doesn't mean you can stop using birth control.)

So although the tests themselves give you legitimate values, I don't think they tell you what you want to know any better than I can from your history and the symptoms you're having.

Making Your HRT Decision

Neither the oestradiol test nor the FSH test will tell you whether you should take oestrogen replacement therapy. Only you and your doctor can decide that, depending on symptoms you may be having, such as hot flushes, night sweats or vaginal dryness, as well as other health concerns, such as your risk of osteoporosis.

Time to Get off the Pill

Q: 'I'm almost 50 years old and thinking of stopping contraceptive pills. I want to see what my periods are like and determine if I'm nearing menopause. How long do I have to stay off the Pill to tell?'

A: *Dr Minkin replies*: You'll have to wait several weeks to see whether or not you get a period and monitor any symptoms, such as hot flushes.

However, the best sign that you've officially reached menopause is when 12 consecutive months have passed without a period.

After you've been off the Pill for several weeks, ask your doctor if he or she will arrange a blood test of your follicle-stimulating hormone (FSH) level to get some idea of where you stand. Keep in mind that your FSH level can fluctuate from day to day as you approach menopause, so one test is not going to give you a sure answer to how close you are to menopause.

TIP: Don't go off contraceptive pills in the summer. 'If you get hot, you won't know if it's due to the weather or hot flushes,' says Dr Minkin. It's best to go off the Pill during the winter months.

Am I There Yet?

Q: 'Since I'm on the Pill and my periods are regular, is there another way to tell whether I'm nearing menopause?'

A: *Dr Minkin replies*: The first clue for most women that they're peri-menopausal (in the transition to menopause) is that their menstrual cycles become irregular. Their periods may occur more often, the flow may be lighter or heavier, or they may begin to skip periods altogether. But in your case, because contraceptive pills are so good at regulating the menstrual cycle, you won't have the benefit of these changes to help guide you. Watch for these signs instead.

Look for Other Clues

During the week you're off the Pill and taking the placebo pills, you may begin to experience symptoms such as hot flushes, night sweats or insomnia. These signs of oestrogen withdrawal occur because you're not getting oestrogen this week, and your body's own oestrogen levels are fluctuating.

Those women who are especially sensitive to changing hormone levels may report headaches during this week as well because without the relaxation effect of oestrogen, blood vessels constrict.

A second way to gauge where you are hormonally is your age. The average age of menopause is 50, so you could simply stop taking the Pill and see what happens. Be sure to use another form of birth control in the meantime. (Note that smoking can accelerate menopause by about two years due to its toxic effect on the ovaries.)

Another test is your mother's age at the time she began menopause. This can be a reliable predictor of when you will go through it, provided that hers was a natural menopause and not the result of a hysterectomy.

Confirming the Menopause

The true sign that you've officially reached menopause is when you've gone without a period for 12 consecutive months. The only way to know this for certain is to stop taking contraceptive pills.

Some women will request that I check their follicle-stimulating hormone (FSH) level with a blood test. (As your ovaries taper off the production of oestrogen, your pituitary gland sends a message to them in the form of a burst of FSH to increase oestrogen production.) A woman's FSH levels can fluctuate enormously during perimenopause, so just a single reading isn't conclusive. But it may give you some indication of where you are. Just make sure you've stopped taking the Pill for at least three to four weeks before the test because it can affect FSH levels and the accuracy of the reading.

But multiple FSH readings over a period of several months are needed for the most accurate results, which your doctor may not be prepared to authorize. In this case, you may wish to go private, but beware of mounting costs! You will have to stop taking contraceptive pills during this time.

A high FSH – one that falls in the range of 40 to 50 mIU/ml (micro international units per millilitre) – especially if you're having hot flushes or night sweats, could mean you're headed in the direction of menopause.

Too Old for Contraceptive Pills?

Q: 'I'm in my fifties and have been experiencing irregular periods, menstrual cramping and other symptoms of perimenopause. My doctor prescribed contraceptive pills. But I'm wondering, am I too old to start taking them?'

A: *Dr Minkin replies*: Today's very low-dose pills, containing just 20 micrograms of oestrogen, are extremely safe for healthy, non-smoking women to use into their early fifties. They ease PMS and menstrual cramps and regulate menstrual changes due to perimenopause. Many women start using the Pill in their forties just to ease irregular bleeding, hot flushes and sleep disturbances.

However, birth control pills don't prevent sexually transmitted diseases and should not be taken if you smoke, have a personal or strong family history of strokes or blood clots, have active liver disease or hepatitis, or have a personal history of breast cancer.

Six Symptoms You Shouldn't Ignore

Q: 'How do I know if my symptoms are caused by menopause, or if I may have a serious disease?'

A: *Toby Hanlon replies:* If you're troubled by hot flushes, missed periods, achy joints and mood swings, don't let your doc send you home with a flip 'It's only the menopause'. It could be something more serious.

When I'm out to dinner with my friends Jill and Helen, 'I don't remember' or 'What's his name?' is a normal part of our conversation. Not surprising for a trio of 50-something women, all of whom can claim to be 'menopausal'. We joke about these 'memory adventures', our 'mature' skin, and 'power surges', as we affectionately call hot flushes.

Tempting as it is to assume that every subtle and not-so-subtle change in your body is just one more thing in this host of menopausal symptoms, in fact they could be signs of something more serious.

'When a woman is of the right age for the menopause, there's almost a knee-jerk reaction on the part of doctors to attribute any symptom to menopause and not investigate other causes,' says Dr James A. Simon, a clinical professor of obstetrics and gynaecology.

This 'go home, it's just the menopause' response is all too common when it comes to women aged 40 to 60, according to Dr Marianne J. Legato, a women's health expert. 'Dismissing or minimizing women's complaints as the menopause or "it's all in your head" puts them at risk of a serious underlying condition going undiagnosed,' explains Dr Legato.

Here's a look at six well-known symptoms associated with the menopause, and how to know when you or your doctor shouldn't write them off as the menopause.

Changes in Periods

Irregular menstrual periods, one of the most common and predictable signs of the menopause, most often occur because of the erratic levels of oestrogen and progesterone and because of less frequent ovulation. Every woman has a unique pattern to her periods and knows what's normal for her. But as you approach the menopause, what's normal can seem to take on a whole new definition.

'We expect periods to become irregular and differ from a woman's usual pattern,' says menopause specialist Jennifer L. Prouty, a registered nurse and chairperson of the consumer education committee for the North American Menopause Society. 'But if something isn't familiar to you and represents a change, you need to see a health provider to check it out,' she warns.

Irregular means periods with bleeding that is lighter or heavier than usual, periods that are closer together, bleeding for fewer or more days than usual, or missed periods altogether.

Keeping a diary to track changes in your menstrual pattern is a good idea so you can see when and where changes occur and tell your doctor, she says.

It May Be the Menopause, But . . .

Menstrual changes that are considered abnormal and need to be checked out include:

- Periods that are very heavy and gushing (flooding), or bleeding with clots
- Periods that last more than seven days, or two or more days longer than usual
- Spotting between periods
- Bleeding after intercourse
- Fewer than 21 days between periods

'Frequently, these symptoms are left unquestioned and untreated for an inordinate amount of time,' says Dr Simon, when in fact they could signal a hormonal imbalance, thyroid disease, uterine fibroids (enlarged by the surge of oestrogen as you approach menopause), uterine polyps (non-cancerous growths in the endometrium), or even cervical or uterine cancer.

Getting the right diagnosis is crucial if you want to avoid unnecessary procedures such as a hysterectomy, says Dr Michelle Warren, medical director of the Center for Menopause, Hormonal Disorders and Women's Health at Columbia University.

Your doctor will want to know what triggers the bleeding and what makes it stop. Tests used to help determine the cause of abnormal bleeding include a smear test; a transvaginal ultrasound, which uses sound waves to visualize the uterus and other pelvic organs with a probe inserted into the vagina; endometrial biopsy, in which a small sample of the uterine lining is removed and examined; and hysteroscopy, where a tiny telescope is inserted into the vagina and through the cervix to look directly at the uterine lining.

Hot Flushes

Hot flushes are the second-most-frequent symptom associated with menopause. When they occur with often drenching perspiration during the night, they're called night sweats.

Hot flushes are the body's way of cooling itself down. Abrupt changes in the body's 'thermostat' in the brain can cause it to mistakenly sense that you're too warm.

So blood vessels dilate and blood rushes to the surface of the skin to cool the body. That's why you get the red, flushed look on your face and neck. Sweating, which sometimes accompanies a hot flush, also cools the body as the perspiration evaporates.

It May Be the Menopause, But . . .

'What I see most frequently misdiagnosed as menopause is hyperthyroidism,' says Dr Warren. That's because its symptoms, which can include flushing, sweating, heat intolerance, heart palpitations and sleeplessness, can easily be confused with those of menopause.

In hyperthyroidism, the thyroid produces excess amounts of the thyroid hormone thyroxine, overstimulating organs as a result and speeding up many of the body's functions. If left untreated, an overactive thyroid can cause a loss of bone mineral density, which, over time, can lead to osteoporosis. Hyperthyroidism can also result in an irregular heartbeat, which can lead to stroke or heart failure.

Unintended weight loss almost always accompanies an overactive thyroid. So if you're losing weight but not dieting, your heart frequently beats rapidly, or you're always hot even when people around you are cold, don't just blame the menopause. 'There's a difference between the intermittent flushing and sweating associated with menopause and being hot and sweating all the time that is not menopause,' cautions Dr Simon.

A simple blood test that measures TSH (thyroid-stimulating hormone) will diagnose hyperthyroidism. (It is more accurate than older tests.) TSH, which is made by the pituitary gland, regulates the amount of thyroid hormone that is released into the blood. When the thyroid gland produces too much thyroid hormone, the pituitary compensates by pumping out less TSH. So a TSH level below normal could be a warning sign.

In some cases, hot flushes and sweating can be indicative of an infectious disease such as tuberculosis, Lyme disease or AIDS. If you also feel sick, your doctor should suspect an infection.

'When you're having menopausal hot flushes, you may feel tired because you haven't had a good night's sleep, but you shouldn't feel sick,' says Dr Simon.

Sweating along with a fever could also be caused by cancer such as leukaemia or lymphomas. A rare tumour of the adrenal gland called a pheochromocytoma and one that usually occurs in the intestine, called a carcinoid tumour, can cause flushing and feelings of warmth, too, which could be mistaken for menopause symptoms.

Hair Loss

'Once a day, I hear "I'm losing my hair. Is it menopause?"' says Dr Minkin. There may well be a connection between dwindling oestrogen levels at menopause and thinning hair, but there's no conclusive data.

It May Be the Menopause, But . . .

It could be a sign of an underactive thyroid, or hypothyroidism. The symptoms are caused by the low levels of thyroxine being produced by the thyroid and circulating through the body. Even subtle changes in thyroid function can affect hair. Complaints of dry skin or brittle nails are also common when the culprit is hypothyroidism.

Women are five times more likely than men to have a thyroid disorder, and it's particularly common as we age. Women between ages 30 and 50 are most typically affected with hypothyroidism, and it's estimated that 10 per cent of women aged 40 and older with the condition go undiagnosed.

Other symptoms of an underactive thyroid also can be easily mistaken for signs of menopause: heavy menstrual bleeding, fatigue, painful joints, mood swings and weight gain. 'Don't let your doctor dismiss these types of symptoms with "What do you expect at your age?"' warns Dr Legato. Ask for a TSH test. That way, you can avoid being given a prescription for oestrogen therapy when you really need a prescription for thyroid hormone. If hypothyroidism is not treated, it can raise your cholesterol and increase your risk of heart disease. It can also lead to a decline in memory and concentration.

Achey Joints

The Japanese don't have a word for hot flushes, but they have one for sore shoulders. Joint pain and stiffness are common but not well-recognized symptoms of menopause, says Dr Warren, because studies have not found a direct link between achey joints and the 'change of life'. 'I see women who have joint pain when they begin having irregular menstrual cycles,' says Jennifer Prouty, 'and I have to wonder if there is a connection.'

We know that a lack of oestrogen affects bone and probably cartilage, too, according to Dr John Klippel, medical director of the Arthritis Foundation. That could explain why osteoarthritis affects mostly women and typically begins when they're in their mid to late forties.

It May Be the Menopause, But . . .

Usually joint pain or stiffness associated with menopause isn't localized to a specific joint but is described more as an overall achiness. The pain and stiffness also don't 'migrate', or occur in your elbow one day and your knee the next.

But pain in key joints such as the hips, knees, lower back or end joints of the fingers is most likely not menopause but osteoarthritis. 'Osteo-arthritis has a pattern to it, so you'll have pain or stiffness when you get up in the morning or after using a joint for a long period of time,' explains Dr Klippel.

See a doctor if the joint pain persists or is accompanied by swelling, or if you have difficulty using the joint. Other causes of joint pain should be ruled out, such as rheumatoid arthritis, fibromyalgia, lupus and Lyme disease.

Depression

'I'm very depressed, and I know it's the menopause' is a complaint that Dr Minkin hears several times a day from her patients.

We know from studies that giving oestrogen to women during peri-menopause (the transition to menopause during which menstrual periods become irregular and hot flushes may start) helps reduce their depression. Other studies have suggested that oestrogen improves mood in post-menopausal women who feel depressed.

But researchers are still trying to work out the relationship between oestrogen and mood. 'There's a growing body of evidence suggesting that neurotransmitters or chemicals in the brain that are associated with mood work better with ample oestrogen and may even require oestrogen to work properly,' explains Dr Simon.

This doesn't mean that depression is inevitable at menopause, but when it does occur, it should be taken seriously and investigated.

It May Be Menopause, But . . .

The most obvious culprits are untreated hot flushes and night sweats. They can leave you feeling irritable and sleep-deprived, which may result in depression and loss of your overall sense of well-being.

Depression can also be a symptom of hypothyroidism. Make sure you've ruled out this condition with a TSH test.

Don't overlook mid-life stresses either. Caring for ageing parents, raising teenagers, career changes or financial problems often hit at this time and can affect anyone's ability to cope. 'There's a tendency for women having other symptoms of oestrogen deficiency, such as hot flushes, night sweats and vaginal dryness, to make the snap judgement that their depression is hormonal and maybe they just need a little oestrogen,' cautions Dr Simon. But a good assessment by your doctor and some soul-searching on your part may reveal that speaking with a mental health professional would be much more beneficial.

Symptoms that go beyond normal feelings of sadness, such as significant changes in weight, social withdrawal, disinterest in life, insomnia, inability to concentrate and anxiety should never be dismissed as 'it's just menopause, and you'll get over it'. You could be experiencing clinical depression, which is best treated with a combination of medication and psychotherapy.

Women with a history of depression seem to be more vulnerable to depression at menopause. So it's especially important for a doctor to recognize the signs so treatment isn't delayed.

Palpitations

Palpitations can feel like the heart is beating erratically or fast, or skipping a beat, or as if there were butterflies in your chest. Usually they occur with hot flushes and night sweats, but they can appear on their own.

'Levels of oestrogen during perimenopause alternate between very high and very low,' says Dr Legato. 'This causes a destabilization of the cardiac rhythm, which can lead to palpitations.'

It May Be the Menopause, But . . .

While palpitations are usually harmless, they could be signs of a serious heart rhythm abnormality or heart disease until proven otherwise.

A revved-up thyroid (hyperthyroidism) can increase the effects of adrenaline, a stress hormone in the body, which can cause a rapid heart rhythm or arrhythmia. It's diagnosed with a TSH test.

Palpitations that occur on a recurring basis in the absence of hot flushes or that are associated with light-headedness or shortness of breath warrant a cardiac evaluation. One test that can be done is an electrocardiogram, called an ECG, which measures the electrical impulses of the heart and can show an irregularity in the heartbeat. (Your doctor may have you wear a portable ECG device called a Holter monitor for 24 hours to record how your heart responds to normal, everyday activities and to determine whether the sensation of palpitations corresponds to a heart rhythm abnormality.) A stress echocardiogram is a very accurate method of diagnosing heart disease in women. It's an imaging technique that combines a treadmill stress test with cardiac ultrasound to check your heart's size, movement, shape and pumping ability.

There's a danger in ascribing palpitations to changing hormone levels. 'When a perimenopausal or menopausal woman says to me, "I'm beginning to experience palpitations", I don't want to brush it off as "just that time of her life" and miss coronary disease,' says Dr Legato.

If it turns out that your palpitations are related to the menopause, they can usually be relieved with oestrogen replacement therapy.

Will Herbs Help You Ease Menopause Symptoms?

Q: 'At the healthfood shop, how do I choose the menopause products that work?'

A: *Dr Minkin replies:* I, too, visited my local healthfood shop recently. The women's nutrition section was filled with various herbal products, all claiming to give your body nutritional and hormonal support for menopause. I know that many women – including my patients – are experimenting on their own with these herbal supplements as an alternative to prescription hormone replacement therapy (HRT) in an effort to eliminate troublesome hot flushes, mood changes and sleep disturbances. But do they really work?

I spoke to Douglas Schar, a London-based clinical herbalist who has a sensible two-step approach for managing symptoms. His advice is to come up with a plan, then take only what you need and only those herbs that we know work. 'Herbal medicine is medicine, and should never be used in a willy-nilly manner,' he cautions.

He prescribes only herbs that have passed his three-part screening process. 'For me to work with a herb,' he explains, 'it must have a substantial history of use, scientific validation that it's effective, and consensus among herbal practitioners that it works.' I asked Doug to share his plan.

Step 1: Hormone Balancing

At menopause, the usual orderly ebb and flow of oestrogen and progesterone becomes erratic, which underlies the symptoms many women experience.

Doug recommends that you choose one of the following hormone-balancing herbs. Although we don't understand exactly how they work, we do know they act on the pituitary gland, ovaries and oestrogen-dependent cells in a way that has been shown in clinical trials to reduce menopausal symptoms. 'I've never had a patient fail to respond to one or the other of these herbs,' he says.

Black Cohosh *(Cimicifuga racemosa)*

Black cohosh is traditionally known as the menopause herb and is one that Doug considers a hormonal treasure chest. It's been shown to be effective at reducing the severity of hot flushes, memory loss, depression and mood swings, and improving the thickness and elasticity of vaginal tissues. Even the American College of Obstetricians and Gynecologists (ACOG) agrees that black cohosh may be an alternative for women who choose not to take HRT.

How much to take: Dried root: two 500-milligram tablets/capsules. Dry standardized extract: follow package instructions for each dose equivalent to 1.5 milligrams of 27-deoxyacteine. Tincture 1:5, 1 teaspoon; tincture 1:1, 20 drops.

How often: Three times a day.

How long: Take it for at least three months to determine if it's working for you. It can be taken as long as you need it.

Cautions: Occasionally causes mild digestive complaints when first taken. Do not use black cohosh in combination with HRT. Women with oestrogen-dependent cancer, including breast, cervical, uterine and ovarian, should consult their doctor before taking it.

Agnus castus *(Vitex or chasteberry)*

Agnus castus, also called vitex or chasteberry, is probably better known as a herb for smoothing out the hormonal ups and downs of the menstrual cycle and premenstrual syndrome (PMS). In Europe, however, it is widely used at menopause.

How much to take: Fruit: two 500-milligram tablets. Dry standardized extract: follow package instructions for each dose equivalent to 250 milligrams of 4:1 chasteberry extract. Tincture 1:5, 60 drops; tincture 1:1, 12 drops.

How often: Twice a day.

How long: Take the herb for at least three months to determine if it's working for you; it can take several months to have the full effect.

TIP: If you experience an unpleasant reaction to a herb, stop taking it immediately.

Step 2: Specific Symptom Relief

Despite taking black cohosh or agnus castus, some women may still have hot flushes, insomnia, mood swings or even heart palpitations. 'It's appropriate to take the next step, which is to choose a herb that specifically targets a breakthrough symptom,' says Doug.

Sage for Hot Flushes

Add common, garden-variety sage to your programme if hot flushes and night sweats persist. It's traditionally used to dry up secretions, including excessive perspiration.

How much to take: As a tea: ½ teaspoon of dried leaf in a mug of boiling water. Tincture 1:1, 20 drops.

How often: Three times a day.

How long: Sage works right away, so use it as needed.

Valerian for Insomnia

Interrupted sleep patterns are very common at menopause. Some women have a hard time falling asleep, wake frequently, or have difficulty falling back to sleep once wakened. Douglas Schar's favourite all-purpose sleep remedy is valerian, which has been shown to help you drift into a deep sleep and stay there.

How much to take: Tincture 1:5, 1 teaspoon in water or juice.

How often: Half an hour before bed.

How long: Valerian works immediately. It can be used for as long as is required to improve sleep patterns.

Cautions: Do not drive after taking valerian because it causes drowsiness. Valerian should not be used while taking sleeping tablets or tranquillizers.

St John's Wort for Depression and Mood Swings

If the blues or mood swings persist, try St John's wort, suggests Doug. It's recognized by the American College of Obstetricians and Gynecologists as helpful for treating mild to moderate depression.

How much to take: Dried herb: two 500-milligram tablets. Dry standardized extract: one 300-milligram tablet standardized to 0.3 per cent hypericin. Tincture 1:5, 1 teaspoon; tincture 1:1, 20 drops.

How often: Three times a day.

How long: You must use this herb continually for four to eight weeks for it to take effect. It can be used long-term.

Cautions: Do not use St John's wort if you are taking any other prescription drugs, without checking with your doctor first. It can cause sensitivity to the sun, so use the strongest sunblock available, and reapply often. If your depression worsens, see your doctor.

Motherwort for Heart Palpitations

Some women experience fluttering or racing sensations of the heart, or palpitations. While benign, they can be alarming the first time you experience them. (Check with your doctor to be sure it's nothing more serious.)

A classic European women's herb called motherwort has been used for centuries. It acts on the nervous system to calm palpitations.

How much to take: Tincture 1:1, 20 drops in water or juice.

How often: Three times a day.

How long: Motherwort is safe to use long-term.

Caution: If you're using any kind of cardiac medication, consult your doctor before taking motherwort.

HRT AND BLACK COHOSH TOGETHER?

Using prescription hormone replacement therapy and black cohosh together is not recommended. 'Both of them work on your endocrine system, so it's best to err on the side of caution. Choose one or the other, but not both,' recommends Douglas Schar, a London-based clinical herbalist.

New Hope for Fibroids?

Q: 'There's a new procedure for fibroids called uterine artery embolization. What is it, and is it safe?'

A: *Dr Minkin replies:* There's a lot of buzz these days about uterine artery embolization, or UAE, because it's 'minimally invasive' and shrinks a fibroid so it doesn't have to be surgically removed. It's being promoted to women as the way to avoid a hysterectomy or myomectomy (surgical removal of the fibroid alone) to relieve troubling symptoms such as pelvic pain and heavy menstrual bleeding.

This makes it an attractive alternative since the majority of hysterectomies are done to treat fibroids. But that argument doesn't automatically mean that UAE is better. Here's a look at what we know and don't know about this procedure.

How UAE Works

UAE is performed by interventional radiologists, specially trained doctors who use x-rays and imaging techniques to see inside the body while they guide narrow catheters or tubes through blood vessels.

UAE shrinks the fibroid by cutting off its blood supply. An incision is made in the groin, and a thin tube called a catheter is inserted into the main artery of the leg. The catheter is guided to each of the uterine arteries, the main source of blood supply to the fibroid. Then polyvinyl alcohol (plastic) particles are injected into the arteries to permanently plug them and prevent blood from 'feeding' the fibroid. All of this is done with the assistance of x-ray images.

Hysterectomy is the only treatment that provides a cure and eliminates the chances that a fibroid will grow back. But the desire to spare the uterus, cut down on hospitalization time and speed recovery has led to the development of other surgical treatments such as myomectomy, which removes just the fibroid, and hysteroscopic resection, which uses electric current to shave off the fibroid inside the uterus and break it into small pieces so it can be removed through the vagina. UAE was developed to provide women with another option and one that did not require surgery.

Effectiveness. Numerous studies conducted since 1997 have shown UAE to be an effective treatment for improving the heavy menstrual bleeding and pelvic pain associated with fibroids.

It has rare serious complications. The most recently published study showed a 58 per cent reduction in fibroid size one year after the procedure, with an improvement in heavy menstrual bleeding and pelvic pressure in 90 per cent of the cases.

Recovery. Expect to stay overnight in the hospital, with total recovery taking one to two weeks. Recovery can be quite painful, and you'll need medication. (The fibroid is dying due to lack of blood flow, which is similar to what happens to the heart muscle during a heart attack.) Some women also experience cramping, nausea, vomiting and low-grade fever for two to seven days after the procedure. This is part of what's called the post-embolization syndrome.

Risks and complications. Studies have found that UAE is very safe and that complications occur in fewer than three per cent of cases. But every medical procedure has risks.

Some of the risks reported for UAE include infection of the uterus, uterine bleeding, premature menopause, persistent pain and reaction to the x-ray imaging material. Complications may result in the need for a hysterectomy.

Unknown factors. UAE is so new that there are no studies of long-term effects, and no studies have directly compared the outcome of UAE with that of any other fibroid treatments. We don't know, for example, if the fibroids will grow back. There are questions concerning the procedure's effect on fertility, which is why it should not be recommended to women who still want to become pregnant. Perhaps the biggest concern is the unknown long-term effects of the plastic particles used to plug up the uterine arteries. They do remain behind and can make their way to other organs.

A special patient registry, sponsored by the Society of Interventional Radiology, the professional organization for interventional radiologists, is collecting information regarding the safety and effectiveness of UAE as well as its effects on fertility and quality of life over the long term in order to answer some of these questions.

Bottom line. The medical establishment currently considers UAE investigational because of the possible serious complications and painful recovery.

I believe it's a step beyond that and has a place among your options for treating fibroids. At this time, however, I'm not a big proponent, largely because of the lack of long-term studies.

It's understandable that doctors become enthusiastic about new procedures, which give their patients more treatment options. But I'm concerned that doctors are marketing UAE to women as their only alternative to a hysterectomy. Believe me, it's not.

FIBROIDS: A VERY COMMON PROBLEM

Fibroids – also called leiomyomas – are a benign overgrowth of the layer of muscle tissue that comprises the uterus. They can range in size from a pea to a cantaloupe melon. Between 25 and 35 per cent of women have fibroids, and for most women, they present no problems. But 10 to 20 per cent of women who have them suffer severe symptoms: heavy menstrual bleeding, pelvic pain and pressure, frequent urination and abdominal distension.

Fibroids are classified by their location within the uterus. Submucosal fibroids lie just under the endometrium, or top layer that lines the uterus, and grow into the uterine cavity; intramural fibroids grow within the uterine muscle wall; and subserosal fibroids grow on the outside wall of the uterus.

Fibroids depend on oestrogen for growth, which is why they're more common in women in their forties, when hormonal changes during perimenopause result in high levels of oestrogen relative to progesterone. This is also the time when they can become symptomatic. The good news is that they shrink after menopause, as long as you don't take oestrogen therapy.

Choosing a treatment that's right for you should be your personal decision, not your doctor's. And a thorough medical evaluation to determine the location, size and number of fibroids is the first step in determining the best course of action for long-term relief.

TIP: Losing weight is one of the best things you can do if you have fibroids. It is well-known that fat tissue produces oestrogen that feeds fibroids.

Ease Worry about Hair Loss

Q: 'I'm self-conscious about my hair, which has been thinning on top since I hit my forties. What can I do?'

A: *Toby Hanlon replies:* You may have female-pattern hair loss, which results in your hair being less dense and finer. Almost half of women in their forties have it, and it's similar to the hair loss that men experience: thinning at the front of the scalp or on the top of the head. But there's no need to panic.

Vive la Différence

'The good news,' says Dr Ellen B. Milstone, clinical associate professor of dermatology at Yale University School of Medicine, 'is that it's very unusual for a woman with female-pattern hair loss to have it progress to the point that she will lose hair all over her head like a man.'

Yet that's most women's biggest fear. So Dr Milstone reassures her patients that the gradual thinning of their hair will level off.

Female-pattern hair loss can also happen early on (when you're in your twenties), though it's more common when women are in their forties. No matter when it occurs, it's best to check with your doctor to rule out other possible causes, such as an overactive or underactive thyroid (hyperthyroidism or hypothyroidism), especially if the hair loss is sudden and more diffuse at the front of the hairline or on the crown.

'A woman in her forties who complains of a gradual thinning over the past few years is more likely experiencing hair loss associated with perimenopause or the onset of menopause,' explains Dr Milstone. (Perimenopause includes the years just before menopause, when a woman begins having irregular menstrual periods and possible hot flushes, and the first year after menopause. Please see 'The Menopause Timeline' on page 12.)

It's not clear just how much dwindling oestrogen levels at menopause contribute to thinning hair. Dr Milstone says that based on her experience, there may be some connection, but there's no conclusive data to support it. 'There are probably multiple causes, not just oestrogen loss,' she speculates.

What You Can Do

Despite your fears, you're not going to lose all of your hair, and this is not a serious medical condition. But since appearance is so important, it's understandable if you're a little upset.

A recent study showed that women who experienced hair loss had feelings of powerlessness, self-consciousness, dissatisfaction with their appearance, embarrassment, frustration at not being able to style their hair the way they wanted, and concern that others would notice.

Darlene Caracappa, who runs a salon that specializes in hair replacement, is often the first person clients meet who can relate to their fears and concerns. 'Most people tell me that their hair is their crowning glory and an important part of who they are,' says Darlene. 'When their hair is depleted, *they* feel depleted.' Women will go to great lengths to work around their hair loss and avoid the fear and embarrassment associated with it. 'They may avoid being outside and exposed to wind or rain, stop going to the gym because sweating makes the hair loss more visible, or get up at 5 am to style their hair,' she explains. But knowing they're not alone and that there *is* a solution is reassuring.

As for the thinning hair itself, Dr Milstone has these suggestions.

- Don't be afraid to wash your hair. It won't lead to further hair loss. (Not washing your hair can lead to dandruff, an itchy scalp and possible trauma from scratching.)

- Avoid brushing or backcombing your hair, which can lead to some hair loss. Comb it instead.

- Try a hairstyle that layers your hair; this will help it look fuller.

- Get a perm or colour your hair if you wish to give it a fuller appearance. Medically, there's no reason not to.

- Consider a hairpiece to add volume to your hair. Avoid hair weaving or extensions, or any other device that can put prolonged tension on your hair or cause the hair to fracture.

What about Regaine (minoxidil), which reportedly increases hair growth and prevents further loss? Dr Milstone says that the 2 per cent strength is minimally, if at all, effective in women, and most women don't want to put a liquid on their scalp twice a day. Besides, it does require continual use to keep the hair that has regrown.

TIP: If you're considering a hairpiece, consult a skilled specialist to help you choose the best option.

Why You Still Need Mammograms

Q: 'I keep hearing that mammograms are ineffectual, but my gynaecologist still recommends them. Do you agree?'

A: *Dr Minkin replies*: A Swedish study recently found that women who had mammograms on a regular basis reduced their risk of dying from breast cancer by 63 per cent. This was encouraging news since previous landmark clinical trials showed the risk to be reduced by 30 per cent.

Around the same time, the British medical journal *The Lancet* published a letter in which two Danish researchers reiterated the original conclusion of a paper they published in 2000 that mammograms are 'unjustified' because there is no reliable evidence that they save lives. If you're like many of my patients, you're probably frustrated, confused and left wondering what to make of all the conflicting information.

For years, doctors, public health officials and women's health advocates have urged women to get mammograms as a means of saving lives through early detection of breast cancer. Is this likely to change now? I'll share my perspective on this and the opinions of several breast cancer experts.

A Flawed Study

In January 2000, two Danish researchers published an analysis of seven randomized trials of mammography screening published in the 1980s and 1990s and concluded that it didn't save lives. (Keep in mind that this was not new research but what is called in scientific lingo 'a secondary analysis of existing data'.) Five of the studies from their analysis were discarded immediately because they were judged to be of poor quality or extremely flawed.

At the time that the analysis was published, it was discredited for being flawed in its own right. 'The Danish researchers made any number of arbitrary decisions and arguable judgements about the quality of the trials,' explains Dr Robert A. Smith, director of cancer screening for the American Cancer Society.

They were very critical of studies that were favourable towards mammography and very accepting of studies that showed no benefit for mammography, according to Dr Smith. The researchers based their conclusion on two studies alone, which is 'just a fraction of the existing world data,' adds Dr Smith. Many experts even wondered how the analysis got published in such a prestigious, peer-reviewed journal as *The Lancet*.

Given all the criticism, last year the Danish researchers reanalysed their findings. To no one's surprise, in a letter they stood by their original conclusion that mammography didn't save lives. This is what made news and led to the latest controversy about mammograms' effectiveness.

What most people didn't realize, however, was that this letter contained no new research findings and was based on their original paper, which had been criticized by many medical and public health experts.

Check the Statistics

'If you approach the issue from a scientific perspective, it's clearly settled,' says Dr Daniel B. Kopans, professor of radiology at Harvard Medical School. Scientists have looked at mammography using the gold standard of research – randomized controlled trials – studies where randomly selected women received the treatment and were compared with women who didn't receive the treatment.

They found a 25 to 30 per cent statistically significant (that is, unlikely to be due to chance) mortality reduction with mammography screening. In addition, many other studies have shown that mammography found breast cancers when they were smaller and at an earlier stage, which we know translates into longer survival. 'In my opinion, these data have not been refuted by the Danish researchers. They just choose not to believe them,' Dr Kopans adds.

The death rate from breast cancer has been steadily dropping by one to two per cent a year since about a decade ago. That's what you'd expect to see, given that mammography screening became more widespread during the mid-1980s, and breast cancer therapy became more effective.

There's no dispute about mammography's value, according to Dr Smith. 'Mammography is a matter of health policy based on a legacy of very strong scientific evidence. The recent analysis by the Danish investigators doesn't change that,' he says.

Women should continue to have confidence in the judgement of numerous US and European groups that have reached a conclusion very different from that of the Danish researchers.

Both Dr Kopans and Dr Smith cite the more recent study in Sweden, which is a much more realistic measure of mammography's lifesaving potential. 'Mammography won't save everyone's life, but as this study demonstrated, it provides the opportunity to reduce the death rate by as much as 63 per cent – twice the benefit previously estimated,' says Dr Kopans.

Still the Best Early Detector

Realistically, no doctor today will tell a woman not to have a mammogram. The truth of the matter is that mammograms are still the best way to find cancer at its earliest stage. 'The tragedy, however, is that there will be women who say that mammography doesn't work, and won't get one,' warns Dr Kopans.

'Four years ago, the average size of a breast cancer detected was two centimetres, or about an inch. Now it is below one centimetre,' says Amy Langer, executive director of the National Alliance of Breast Cancer Organizations and a 17-year breast cancer survivor. She attributes this to early detection and the vastly improved quality of mammograms today.

Given what we know about the biology of breast cancer, when there's a smaller lesion, the chance of treating it successfully goes up. 'It's the difference between fighting a war against 10,000 adversaries versus 100,000,' Amy Langer adds. But the benefits of mammography aren't just about finding breast cancer. 'It is never unnecessary to know that you *don't* have breast cancer,' she says.

Finding breast cancer early also affects your treatment choices. This is something that tends to be ignored by studies that measure mammography's worth only in terms of death rates.

The quality of a woman's life is important and if tumours can be detected at an earlier stage, when it can be treated with a lumpectomy rather than mastectomy, or when a patient won't need radiation or chemotherapy, it can make a huge difference in her life.

Mammography isn't perfect. It doesn't find breast cancer 100 per cent of the time. Sometimes it finds abnormalities that a biopsy later shows aren't cancer. But its limitations just mean that we have to continue looking for better ways to detect breast cancer earlier, develop treatments that can reverse it, and even find ways to prevent it.

The message to women and their healthcare providers is that the Danish study doesn't alter the fact that the preponderance of data clearly shows a benefit.

The debate about mammography may never be settled to everyone's satisfaction. In the meantime, says Amy Langer, don't forgo the opportunity to have the biggest edge against breast cancer you can by doing what is within your control. 'You can't pick your genes or your parents' but you can do everything in your power to make sure you find breast cancer if it's there.'

We recommend this schedule of mammogram screenings.

- Regular mammograms starting at the of age 50

- Annual clinical breast examination by a trained professional

- Monthly breast self-examination

Currently, the Breast Screening Programme provides free breast screening every three years for all women in the UK aged 50 and over, although only those up to the age of 64 are routinely invited. Breast screening is offered free for women aged 50 to 69 in Australia, and in New Zealand for women aged 50 to 64. In South Africa, there is no consensus on the policy of using mammography and women are left to make up their own minds. The big question for many women is whether their medical insurance will pay for it, and the answer will undoubtedly influence their decision. If you are worried about the infrequency of the scans, or the late age at which they start, you can pay for scans to be undertaken privately.

Wind and the Hormone Connection

Q: 'Now that I'm having perimenopausal symptoms, I've also started developing embarrassing wind. Is there a connection?'

A: *Dr Minkin replies*: We know that sex-related hormones like oestrogen do have an effect on gastrointestinal activity. Many women, for example, become constipated just before their periods and then have looser stools once their periods begin. This is thought to be related to changing levels of oestrogen and progesterone during the menstrual cycle.

Premenopausal women also have what is known as slower gastric emptying and transit time than men, possibly due to oestrogen. This means that food and liquids tend to move more slowly through their gastrointestinal tracts.

When it comes to the menopause, however, there's no evidence as yet that decreasing levels of oestrogen result in an increase in wind. Dr Lin Chang, a gastroenterologist at UCLA School of Medicine, has compared complaints of bloating (typically due to gas) in premenopausal and postmenopausal women with irritable bowel syndrome.

She found little difference in bloating symptoms between the two groups. 'There are hormonal and age-related influences on gut function in terms of sensation and transit time,' explains Dr Chang. 'But the effects of the menopause on symptoms of wind and bloating have not been well-studied.'

Possible Culprits

It's difficult to pin down any one reason why some women experience a 'wind crisis' with the menopause. Dr Chang and her colleague, Dr Margaret Heitkemper, offer some theories.

- Since oestrogen appears to slow the rate at which the stomach empties and food moves through the small intestines, the decrease in oestrogen at menopause could speed up both of these, perhaps leading to more wind and bloating.

- As we age and the activity of our colons slows down, constipation increases. (It's possible that changes in parts of the nervous system that regulate bowel function are affected by ageing.) More constipation could mean more wind and bloating. Slower colon transit time could also mean that less wind is expelled, resulting in bloating.

- An underlying condition – such as lactose intolerance, chronic constipation or irritable bowel syndrome – can precipitate an increase in wind or a change in transit time, or it can lead to an enhanced perception of and sensitivity to wind.

- Women at mid-life may be trying to eat a more healthy diet of fruit, vegetables and whole grains, which could increase wind.

- What you may think is wind could be fluid retention and premenstrual bloating (both very common during perimenopause due to hormonal imbalances).

No More 'Oops, Excuse Me!'

Here are suggestions from Dr Chang and Dr Heitkemper that should help with the wind and bloating.

- Evaluate your diet to see if you are eating more high-fibre and wind-producing foods than usual, such as beans, vegetables and fruit. Increase fibre intake gradually to avoid this.

- Check for lactose intolerance. Try eliminating all dairy products for two weeks. Then add them back, and see if symptoms return. If they do, eat the foods in smaller amounts, include them in meals, switch to lactose-free products, or try lactose enzyme tablets that help digest milk sugar. (You can probably eat yoghurt with live and cultures and experience few symptoms.)

- Eliminate or reduce the number of sugar-free foods you eat. They are sweetened with sorbitol, which can give some people wind.

- Decrease gum chewing and the use of straws, which increase the amount of air you ingest.

Persistent bloating that is not associated with your menstrual cycle should be evaluated by a doctor; it could be a sign of a more serious health problem, such as ovarian cancer. If chronic constipation is a problem, or if you're experiencing symptoms of irritable bowel syndrome (recurrent or chronic abdominal discomfort, alternating constipation and diarrhoea), see a doctor.

TIP: Give your diet (and colon) a fibre boost by trading your cornflakes for sultana bran.

'Moisturize My *What*?'

Q: 'I have atrophic vaginitis. Is this an infection?'

A: *Dr Minkin replies*: Atrophic vaginitis, or vaginal atrophy, is not an infection but a result of declining hormone levels most often seen at menopause. The delicate tissues of the vagina become thinner and drier. Low oestrogen can also cause the vagina to narrow and shorten, or atrophy. These changes can lead to irritation, inflammation and painful intercourse. Here's what you can do.

Treat the Cause

Replacing lost oestrogen will treat the underlying cause of vaginal atrophy by increasing the natural moisture of the vagina as well as blood flow, making it easier for the vagina to lubricate itself.

Oral oestrogen replacement therapy will treat vaginal atrophy as well as other symptoms of menopause, such as hot flushes. But you can also just treat the problem 'locally' with these forms of oestrogen.

- Vaginal oestrogen creams such as Premarin and Ovestin – or the newer tablet, called Vagifem – are inserted into the vagina and absorbed directly by the vaginal tissues.

- A vaginal ring called Estring is worn in the vagina and releases a continuous dose of oestrogen for three months.

Treat the Symptoms

If you want a hormone-free solution, try an over-the-counter personal lubricant or vaginal moisturizer. Lubricants are used during sex and coat the vagina. Examples include Astroglide and KY Jelly. (Orgasms naturally help lubricate the vagina by increasing blood supply.)

Vaginal moisturizers, on the other hand, act directly on vaginal tissue to replenish and maintain moisture. Their effects typically last for days, and they are most effective when used on a regular schedule. Brands include Replens, Vagisil Intimate Moisturizer, Astroglide, Australian Bodycare Hormone-free Vaginal Moisturizer and Durex Sensilube.

Make Peace with Your 'Pot'

Q: 'I have a little bubble of fat between my navel and pubic bone. It was there even when I worked out five times a week and weighed 10 stone. Is it something I'm eating that's causing it, or is there a genetic reason for why I have this "paunch"?'

A: *Dr Peeke replies*: The 'paunch' is an inevitable part of middle age. I have my own names for this phenomenon. It's 'menopot' for women and 'manopot' for men.

As we get older, especially after age 40, we accumulate more fat under the skin in the lower part of the abdomen. It's usually about 2 to 3.5 kg (5 to 8 lb) of fat that lies above the abdominal muscle wall. The fat's not associated with any significant illness or death, but if you accumulate too much of it under the abdominal muscle wall, deep inside the tummy, that's a whole different matter. Too much fat deep inside is toxic weight, which is highly associated with increased risk of heart disease, high blood pressure, diabetes and cancer.

You can tell the difference between the two types of fat by lying flat on your back on the floor. If your abdomen rises well above your front pelvic bones, as it would in a pregnancy, you have toxic weight. A menopot or manopot, on the other hand, will tend to flatten out and fall to the side, because the fat is external. So make peace with your pot, but get rid of any toxic weight.

RESOURCES

Amarant Trust (Menopause)
This charity helps women deal with problems they might experience during the
menopause. Excellent information, resources and support.
Gainsborough Clinic
22 Barkham Terrace
Lambeth Road
London SE1 7PW
Helpline: 01293 413000 (11am–6pm)
www.amarantmenopausetrust.org.uk

Breast Cancer Care
Provider of information, practical assistance and emotional support for anyone
affected by breast cancer.
Kiln House
210 New King's Road
London SW6 4NZ
Tel: 020 7384 2984
Helpline: 0800 800 6000
Email: bcc@breastcancercare.org.uk
www.breastcancercare.org.uk

Breast Cancer Campaign
Breast Cancer Campaign funds independent breast cancer research throughout the
UK. Information about breast cancer, how to check your breasts and the latest
news on research.
Clifton Centre
110 Clifton Street
London EC2A 4HT
www.bcc-uk.org

The British Wheel of Yoga

Recognized by Sport England as the governing body for yoga in Great Britain.
Central Office
25 Jermyn Street
Sleaford, Lincs
NG34 7RU
Tel: 01529 306851
Fax: 01529 303233
Email: office@bwy.org.uk

CancerBACUP

Europe's leading cancer information service, with the latest recources, practical
advice and support for cancer patients, their families and carers.
3 Bath Place
Rivington Street
London EC2A 3JR
Helpline: 0808 800 1234
www.cancerbacup.org.uk

Cancer Research UK

The world's largest independent organization dedicated to cancer research.
PO Box 123
Lincoln's Inn Fields
London WC2A 3PX
Tel: (Customer Services) 020 7009 8820
Tel: (Switchboard) 020 7242 0200
Fax: 020 7269 3100
www.cancerresearchuk.org

The Daisy Network

Support group specifically for women with premature menopause.
PO Box 183
Rossendale BB4 6WZ
Email: info@daisynetwork.org.uk
www.daisynetwork.org.uk

Endometriosis Society
Provides information and support to women with endometriosis.
Suite 50, Westminster Palace Gardens
1-7 Artillery Row
London SW1P 1RL
Helpline: 0808 808 2227
Tel: 020 7222 2781
Email: nes@endo.org.uk
www.endo.org.uk

Fibroid Embolisation
Gives the latest information on the condition, as well as details on the various
forms of treatment.
The Department of Radiology
The Royal Surrey County Hospital
Egerton Road
Guildford
Surrey GU2 5XX
Tel: 01483 464053
www.fibroids.co.uk

British Thyroid Foundation
Charity dedicated to helping those with thyroid disorders, supporting both patients
and their families.
PO Box 97
Clifford
Wetherby
West Yorkshire LS23 6XD
Tel: 0870 7707933
www.btf-thyroid.org

Hysterectomy Association
Provides impartial advice on hysterectomy and its long-term health implications.
60 Redwood House
Charlton Down
Dorchester DT2 9UH
Tel: 0871 781 1141
www.hysterectomy-association.org.uk

Medical Research Council
The MRC is a government-funded body involved in medical research, including clinical trials and research into cancer.
www.mrc.ac.uk

National Osteoporosis Society
The National Osteoporosis Society (NOS) is a UK national charity dedicated to eradicating osteoporosis and promoting bone health in both men and women.
Camerton
Bath BA2 0PJ
Helpline: 01761 472721
www.nos.org.uk

Ovacome (Ovarian Cancer)
Support and advice for ovarian cancer sufferers.
St Bartholomew's Hospital
West Smithfield
London EC1A 7BE
Tel: 020 7600 5141
Email: ovacome@ovacome.org.uk

Royal College of Obstetricians and Gynaecologists
The RCOG is dedicated to the encouragement of the study and the advancement of the science and practice of obstetrics and gynaecology.
27 Sussex Place
Regent's Park
London NW1 4RG
Tel: 020 7772 6200 (general enquiries)
www.rcog.org.uk

Women's Health
Women's Health publishes health information booklets on gynaecological and sexual health issues.
52 Featherstone Street
London EC1Y 8RT
Office tel: 020 7251 6333
Health enquiry line: 0845 125 5254
Email: health@womenshealthlondon.org.uk
www.womenshealthlondon.org.uk

Women's Nutrition Advisory Service
A fantastic resource for women, dealing with nutrition for all ages and health
conditions.
PO Box 268
Lewes
East Sussex
BN7 1QN
Tel: 01273 487366
Email: wnas@wnas.org.uk

AUSTRALIAN CONTACTS

Australian College of General Practitioners
The professional body for general practitioners in Australia. The College provides
news on current medical treatments, including hormone replacement therapy.
RACGP College House
1 Palmerston Crescent
South Melborne VIC 3205
Tel: 03 8699 0414
www.racgp.org.au

Australian Menopause Society
This organization aims to encourage research and scientific discussion of the
menopause, and promote understanding through information and education.
Their website includes listings for doctors, various resources including self-
assessment tests for menopause-related health problems and information leaflets,
and details of scientific studies currently being conducted.
AMS Secretariat
PO Box 1228
Buderim QLD 4556
Tel: 07 5456 2660
Fax: 07 5456 2661
www.menopause.org.au

Australian Women's Health Network
Community-based advocacy, information and lobbying organization. The network provides information relating to a variety of women's health issues.
c/o Dr Helen Keleher
29/219 Auburn Road
Hawthorn VIC 3122
Tel: 03 9244 6688
Fax: 03 9244 6017
www.awhn.org.au

Beyond Blue
Australia's national depression initiative, Beyond Blue provides access to resources, information and research relating to depression.
50 Burwood Road
PO Box 6100
Hawthorn VIC 3122
Tel: 03 9810 6100
www.beyondblue.org.au

Breasthealth
Online resources service providing information for women with breast cancer and their partners, family members and friends. The website includes information on diagnosis, types of breast cancer, treatments, emotional effects and support, and a glossary.
www.breasthealth.com.au

Breastscreen Australia
Australia's national mammographic screening programme. Breastscreen Australia provides free mammograms to women between the ages of 50-69.
Tel: 13 20 50 (Australia-wide)
www.breastscreen.info.au

The Cancer Council Australia
Australia's national non-government cancer control organization. Provides information about cancer and cancer prevention.
www.cancer.org.au

Cervical Screening
Australia's national cervical screening campaign.
www.cervicalscreen.health.gov.au

Depression Information Resource
Online resources for people living with depression and their family and friends.
www.depressionet.com.au

Endometriosis Association
The EA provides information and resources relating to endometriosis and runs
support groups for women with the condition. There are branches in all states.
567 Waterdale Road
Heidelberg West VIC 3081
Tel: 03 9457 2933
Email: info@endometriosis.org.au

Health Insite
Australian Government initiative providing access to information about health
from health organizations, government agencies and educational and research
institutions. Includes resources relating specifically to the menopause.
www.healthinsite.gov.au

The Jean Hailes Foundation
Women's health organization providing clinical care, education and research.
PO Box 1108
Clayton South VIC 3169
Australia
Tel: 03 9562 6771 (Education) or 03 9543 9612 (Research Unit)
www.jeanhailes.org.au

Nutrition Australia
Non-governmental community-based organization that provides information on
nutrition.
The Exercise Science and Rehabilitation Centre
University of Wollongong
Northfields Avenue
Wollongong NSW 2522
Tel: 02 4221 5346
Fax: 02 4221 5717
www.nutritionaustralia.org

Osteoporosis Australia
This organization provides information and education about osteoporosis for the
public and healthcare professionals.
Level 1, 52 Parramatta Road
Forest Lodge NSW 2037
Tel: 02 9518 8140
www.osteoporosis.org.au

**Royal Australian and New Zealand College of Obstetricians and
Gynaecologists**
Professional body providing training and accreditation for obstetricians and
gynaecologists in Australia and New Zealand, as well as research and advocacy in
related fields.
College House
254–260 Albert St
East Melbourne VIC 3002
Tel: 03 9417 1699
www.ranzcog.edu.au

New Zealand Contacts

New Zealand Government Online
Access any New Zealand government site, including many health sites.
www.govt.nz

New Zealand Breast Cancer Foundation
Charitable trust that provides information on breast cancer.
PO Box 99 650
Newmarket
Auckland
Tel: 09 308 0243
Fax: 09 308 0244
TelstraClear Toll Free: 0800 902 732
www.nzbcf.org.nz

Cancer Society of New Zealand

This not-for profit organization provides information about cancer, support for cancer patients and their families, advocacy and programmes aimed at reducing the incidence and risk of cancer. Also provides major research funding.
PO Box 10847
Wellington
Tel: 04 494 7270
Fax: 04 494 7271
www.cancernz.org.nz

Everybody

(formerly NZ Health Online)
New Zealand-based consumer health resource.
www.everybody.co.nz/cc

Healthy Women

The national cervical screening and mammographic programme. Includes information and advice on breast and cervical cancer, and the screening process.
PO Box 92 522
Wellesley Street
Auckland
Tel: 09 580 9000
Fax: 09 580 9001
www.healthywomen.org.nz

Mental Health Commission

Government body responsible for monitoring key mental health agencies and working with the sector to promote understanding of mental illness. Provides information and access to resources.
www.mhc.govt.nz

Mental Health Foundation

The Mental Health Foundation provides information about mental health issues and help accessing relevant support and resources.
81 New North Road
Eden Terrace
Auckland
Tel: 09 300 7010
Fax: 09 300 7020
www.mentalhealth.org.nz

Osteoporosis New Zealand
Provides information, education, advocacy and resources relating to osteoporosis
and bone health.
Osteoporosis New Zealand Inc
P O Box 688
Wellington
Tel: 04 499 4862
Fax: 04 499 4863
www.bones.org.nz

Women's Health Action
Women's health advocacy group.
PO Box 9947
Newmarket
Auckland
Tel: 09 520 5295
Fax: 09 520 5731
www.womens-health.org.nz

RECOMMENDED READING

Abensur, Nadine. *The Cranks Bible: A Timeless Collection of Vegetarian Recipes.* Weidenfeld, 2002.

Clark, Jan. *Hysterectomy and the Alternatives.* Vermilion, 2000.

Clark, Jane. Jane Clarke's *Bodyfoods Cookbook: Recipes for Life.* Weidenfeld, 2001.

Elliot, Rose. *The Bean Book: Essential Vegetarian Collection.* HarperCollins, 2000.

Glenville, Marilyn. *New Natural Alternatives to HRT.* Kyle Cathie, 2003.

Glenville, Marilyn. *Eat Your Way Through the Menopause.* Kyle Cathie, 2002.

Humphries, Carolyn. *The Classic 1000 Vegetarian Recipes.* Foulsham, 2002.

Lee, John R. *Premenopause: What Your Doctor May Not Tell You.* Little Brown, 1999.

Lee, John R. and Virginia Hopkins. *What Your Doctor May Not Tell You About Menopause: Breakthrough Book on Natural Progesterone.* Little Brown, 1996.

Leneman, Leah. *The Tofu Cookbook: Over 150 Quick and Easy Recipes.* HarperCollins, 1998.

Maddern, Jan. *Yoga Builds Bones.* Fair Weather Press, 2002.

Maleskey, Gale and Mary Kittel. *The Hormone Connection: How Hormones Affect Women's Health and How to Achieve a Better Hormone Balance.* Rodale, 2003.

Marks, Betty. *High Calcium Low Calorie Cookbook.* Publishers Group West, 2003.

Murray, Jenni. *Is It Me or Is It Hot in Here?: A Modern Woman's Guide to the Menopause.* Vermilion, 2003.

Plant, Jane. *Your Life in Your Hands: Understanding, Preventing and Overcoming Breast Cancer.* Virgin Books, 2003.

Plant, Jane and Gill Tidey. *Understanding, Preventing and Overcoming Osteoporosis.* Virgin Books, 2003.

Stewart, Maryon. *The Phyto Factor: A Revolutionary Way to Boost Overall Health – Reducing the Risk of Cancer, Heart Disease and Osteoporosis – And to Control the Menopause Naturally.* Vermilion, 2000.

Stoppard, Miriam. Menopause: *The Complete Guide to Maintaining Health and Well-being and Managing Your Life.* Dorling Kindersley, 2001

Weed, Susun S. *New Menopausal Years: The Wise Woman Way.* Ash Tree Publishing, 2002.

West, Dr Christine. *Family Doctor Guide to Hysterectomy & The Alternatives.* Dorling Kindersley, 2000.

USING HERBS AND SUPPLEMENTS SAFELY

While herbs are generally safe and cause few, if any, side effects, you should use them responsibly. Above all, if you are under a doctor's care for any health condition or are taking any drugs, don't take any herb without your doctor knowing about it. Certain natural substances can change the way your body absorbs and processes certain medications.

Every product has the potential to cause adverse reactions. Below are cautions for the herbs mentioned in this book that may be more likely than others to cause adverse reactions in some people. Though such occurrences are rare, you should be aware of what they are and discontinue use of the herb if you experience an unusual reaction. Also, do not exceed the recommended dosages: more is *not* better. And consult a qualified medical herbalist if you are considering taking more than one herb at a time.

HERB	SAFE USE GUIDELINES AND POSSIBLE SIDE EFFECTS
Agnus castus (also known as vitex or chasteberry) *(Vitex agnus-castus)*	May counteract the effectiveness of birth control pills. Do not use during pregnancy.
Alfalfa *(Medicago sativa)*	Safe.
Angelica sinensis (also known as dong quai) *(Angelica sinensis)*	Generally regarded as safe.
Asian ginseng *(Panax ginseng)*	May cause irritability if taken with caffeine or other stimulants. Do not take if you have high blood pressure.
Black cohosh *(Actea racemosa)*	Do not use for more than six months.

HERB	SAFE USE GUIDELINES AND POSSIBLE SIDE EFFECTS
Black haw *(Viburnum prunifolium)*	Do not take without medical supervision if you have a history of kidney stones as it contains oxalates, which can cause kidney stones.
Black tea *(Camellia sinensis)*	Black tea is not recommended for excessive or long-term use because it can stimulate the nervous system.
Chamomile *(Matricaria recutita)*	Very rarely can cause an allergic reaction when ingested. People allergic to closely related plants such as ragweed, asters and chrysanthemums should drink the tea with caution.
Cinnamon *(Cinnamomum zeylanicum)*	Generally regarded as safe.
Cramp bark *(Viburnum opulus)*	Generally regarded as safe.
Damiana *(Turnera diffusa;* *T. aphrodisiaca)*	Generally regarded as safe.
Dandelion leaves *(Taraxacum officinale)*	If you have high blood pressure, see your doctor first before trying dandelion.
Dandelion root *(Taraxacum officinale)*	If you have gallbladder disease, do not use dandelion root preparations without medical approval. If you have high blood pressure, see your doctor first before trying dandelion.
Echinacea *(Echinacea, spp.)*	Do not use if allergic to closely related plants such ragweed, asters and chrysanthemums. Do not use if you have tuberculosis or an autoimmune condition such as lupus or multiple sclerosis because echinacea stimulates the immune system.
False unicorn root (also known as Helonias) *(Chamaelirium luteum)*	May cause nausea and vomiting in doses higher than five to 15 drops of tincture or 125 ml of infusion. Do not use during pregnancy.
Fenugreek *(Trigonella foenum-graecum)*	Generally regarded as safe.
Garlic *(Allium sativum)*	Do not use supplements if you're on anti-coagulants or before undergoing surgery because garlic thins the blood and may increase bleeding. Do not use if you're taking drugs to lower your blood sugar.
Ginger *(Zingiber officinale)*	May increase bile secretion, so if you have gallstones, do not use therapeutic amounts of the dried root or powder without guidance from a doctor.

HERB	SAFE USE GUIDELINES AND POSSIBLE SIDE EFFECTS
Green tea *(Camellia sinensis)*	Generally regarded as safe.
Guggul *(Commiphora mukul)*	Rarely, may trigger diarrhoea, restlessness, apprehension or hiccups. Do not use during pregnancy.
Helonias *(Chamaelirium luteum)*	See False unicorn.
Horsetail *(Equisetum* spp.)	Do not use the tincture if you have heart or kidney problems. May cause a thiamin deficiency. Do not take more than two grams per day of powdered extract or take for prolonged periods. Do not use if you're taking hypoglycaemic drugs.
Lady's mantle *(Alchemilla vulgaris)*	Generally considered safe.
Liquorice root *(Glycyrrhiza glabra)*	Do not use if you have diabetes, high blood pressure, liver or kidney disorders or low potassium levels. Do not use daily for more than four to six weeks because overuse can lead to water retention, high blood pressure caused by potassium loss, or impaired heart and kidney function. Do not use during pregnancy.
Milk thistle seed *(Silybum marianum)*	Generally considered safe.
Motherwort *(Leonurus cardiaca)*	Generally considered safe. Do not use during pregnancy.
Nettle *(Urtica dioica)*	If you have allergies, your symptoms may worsen, so take only one dose a day for the first few days.
Oat straw *(Avena sativa)*	Do not use if you have coeliac disease (gluten intolerance) as it contains gluten, a grain protein.
Partridgeberry *(Mitchella repens)*	Generally considered safe.
Peppermint *(Mentha piperita)*	Generally considered safe.
Red clover *(Trifolium pratense)*	Generally considered safe.
Rose *(Rosa* spp.)	Generally considered safe.
Sage *(Salvia officinalis)*	Used in therapeutic amounts, can increase sedative side-effects of drugs. Do not use if you're hypoglycaemic or undergoing anti-convulsant therapy. Generally considered safe when used as a spice.

HERB	SAFE USE GUIDELINES AND POSSIBLE SIDE EFFECTS
St John's wort *(Hypericum perforatum)*	Do not use with antidepressants or other prescription medicine without medical approval. May cause photosensitivity; avoid overexposure to direct sunlight.
Sarsaparilla *(Smilax spp.)*	May speed elimination of prescription medications thereby requiring an increase in the effective dose.
Siberian ginseng (also known as Eleuthero) *(Eleutherococcus senticosus)*	Generally considered safe.
Skullcap *(Scutellaria laterifolia)*	Generally considered safe.
True unicorn root *(Aletris farinosa)*	May cause a drug interaction with some oxytocin drugs.
Turmeric *(Curcuma domestica)*	Do not use as a home remedy if you have high stomach acid or ulcers, gallstones or bile duct obstruction. Do not use during pregnancy.
Valerian *(Valeriana officinalis)*	Do not use with sleep-enhancing or mood-regulating medications because it may intensify their effects. May cause heart palpitations and nervousness in sensitive individuals. If such stimulant action occurs, discontinue use.
Vitex *(Vitex agnus-castus)*	See agnus castus.
Wild yam *(Dioscorea villosa)*	Generally considered safe.
Yellow dock root *(Rumex crispus)*	If you have a history of kidney stones, do not take without medical supervision as it contains oxalates and tannins, which may adversely affect this condition.

INDEX

Bold type indicates boxed text; *italics* indicate illustrations or tables.

OTHER RODALE BOOKS

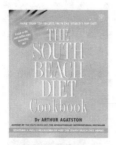
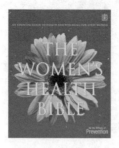
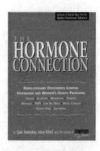
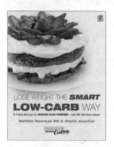
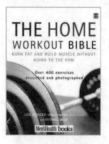
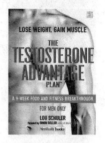
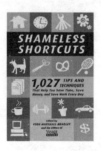
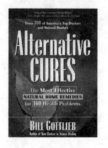
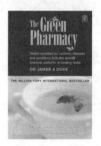

Visit our website **www.rodalestore.co.uk** or to place an order call

UK 0800 7310 6222
South Africa 011 265 4311
Australia 1800 077 550
New Zealand 0800 442 384

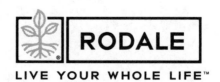